8/... ...4/19

D0362389

RAPID
FITNESS

RAPID
FITNESS

ELEVATE YOUR FITNESS TO NEW HEIGHTS IN MINUTES

ZEN MARTINOLI

JOHN BLAKE

Published by John Blake Publishing Ltd,
3 Bramber Court, 2 Bramber Road,
London W14 9PB, England

www.johnblakepublishing.co.uk

www.facebook.com/johnblakebooks
twitter.com/jblakebooks

This edition published in 2015

ISBN: 978 1 78418 119 2

British Library Cataloguing-in-Publication Data:

A catalogue record for this book is available from the British Library.

Design by www.envydesign.co.uk

Printed in Great Britain by CPI Group (UK) Ltd

1 3 5 7 9 10 8 6 4 2

Papers used by John Blake Publishing are natural, recyclable products made
from wood grown in sustainable forests. The manufacturing processes
conform to the environmental regulations of the country of origin.

Every attempt has been made to contact the relevant copyright-holders,
but some were unobtainable. We would be grateful if the appropriate
people could contact us.

ACKNOWLEDGEMENTS

Firstly I want to thank the photographer Michele Martinoli for shooting and producing all the images for the book. The incredible amount of work and time invested is greatly appreciated.

A special thank you also to…

Lisa Mudie for her time, patience and being a brilliant model in the book and on the cover – and a great friend.

Jason Van Veldhuysen for his expertly written foreword and overall support of both *Rapid Fitness* and *5 Minute Fitness*.

Ade Adelano (Everlast UK Licensee) for his continued support and sponsorship.

Chris, Ray and the team and John Blake Publishing for embracing my ideas and publishing them!

Contact Zen Martinoli on:

Instagram: @rapid_fitness
Email: zen@thefitnessfighter.com
zen@rapid-fitness.net

www.rapid-fitness.net – a dedicated site containing a
database of all of the exercise images found in this book.

www.thefitnessfighter.com

CONTENTS

FOREWORD

The biggest factor in any successful fitness program is motivation. If you can't get psyched up to tackle the exercises and perform the work, your program won't take you very far. In my experience, motivation is enhanced by the overall effectiveness of the program, the variety and enjoyment of performing the exercises and the results of your labour. You may bring to the table a strong work ethic and desire to achieve your goals but, without the factors just mentioned, you will quickly look to a new program.

In my own personal pursuits – as a former competitive boxer who has moved into coaching, entrepreneurship and fatherhood – I struggle with time constraints and its effect on my athletic output. After a full day of work, spending time with family and working with fighters, finding the motivation to train is more of a challenge than ever. My main focus regarding performance is how to get the most out of my workouts in less than half the time and still maintain a competitive edge over my peers, earning the respect of my fighters. Not only do I prepare fighters for one of the most difficult tasks of their lives, but I myself step in the ring with them on occasion to develop their skills and show them what it takes to win.

In the past year I have worked with Zen to integrate his methods and workout combinations into my routine. I've increased my agility and explosiveness in the ring, as well as my overall athletic capabilities. This has offset the decline in my actual boxing skills, since I don't have hours each day to refine my punches and footwork. I can only imagine what I'd have been able to achieve had I been working with Zen when I was competing, nine years ago.

From the perspective of a coach, I'm always looking for the newest, most effective training methods and have integrated Zen's workout routines into the program design for my fighters. Since boxing is such a skill-oriented sport, a lot of time is spent working partner drills, sparring and drilling at specific boxing stations. As a result, any time devoted to conditioning has to be highly effective and intelligently used; there isn't a moment or a burst of energy to waste. It all has to hit the bottom line and optimally prepare fighters for the intensity of a boxing match.

We have seen a revolution in the fitness industry over the past ten years due to the accessibility of online information. Anybody can look up how to perform fundamental strength-training exercises and get a basic understanding of how to approach fitness. Aspiring athletes can get an inside look at how the top performers in their chosen sport are training. This has resulted in both positive and negative effects: on one hand, the bar has been raised; after a number of months in the gym, coupled with online research, the average fitness enthusiast acquires a basic set of knowledge on par with that of trainers around for ten years. Yet on the other hand, there is such an overload of information that they struggle to organise exercises and routines that yield results beyond the basic level.

If you are looking to break through plateaus, or trying to make the most of limited time and equipment, *Rapid Fitness* is your gateway to cutting-edge, scientific training. In this book, Zen outlines a variety of short, intelligent workouts designed to shock your system, keep you motivated and push you to new levels. Use this book as a way to synthesize your current workout routines, or to address weak areas. If you are seeking to improve your vertical jump, agility, or explosive strength, start with routines that tackle those weaknesses. Read the book through quickly the first time and then start to pick out what will motivate you and give you the best results. From there, you have almost limitless options.

Jason Van Veldhuysen, author of *Beginner Boxing: A Roadmap to Your First Fight*, Toronto, Canada.
www.precisionstriking.ca

CHAPTER ONE

INTRODUCTION TO RAPID FITNESS AND THE RAPID-WORKOUT

Important: these programs are not suitable for beginners. A solid fitness background is required before taking part. If you are untrained, sedentary, or have underlying health problems or biomechanical issues, it is inadvisable to participate at this level of activity, as there is an increased risk of injury.

When used correctly these workouts will amplify your performance levels, engendering improvements in speed, strength and power. This chapter will explain the methodology behind the rapid-workouts, their application and physiological benefits. It is important to note that, due to the high intensity of the workouts, they should be 'cycled' properly with adequate breaks. Recommendations for program structure are made to ensure your continued progress. It is imperative that you have a sufficient aerobic base before you attempt any of the HIIT (High-Intensity Interval Training) routines, as well as existing muscular integrity to perform the exercises. It is also prudent to identify any muscular imbalances that you may have before embarking on the workouts, as failure to do so may lead to injury and compromise your progress. In addition, orthopaedic screening is advised to identify any biomechanical impediments.

Welcome to *Rapid Fitness*, an essential companion for recreational exercisers and sportspeople on the go.

No gym? No time? No problem!
Contained within are a collection of short, convenient, high-intensity – or 'rapid' – workouts intended for men and women who have already achieved a significant level of fitness.[1]

The rapid-workouts, which typically last between five and fifteen minutes, can be employed anywhere at any time, require no equipment and use bodyweight only (a stopwatch will be required for timed workouts). They are specifically designed to deliver improvements to both your aerobic [2] and anaerobic fitness.[3] These mostly 'compound' (multi-joint) bodyweight movements provide all the benefits associated with functional fitness,[4] enhancing your speed, strength, power, endurance, flexibility, motor skills, co-ordination and core strength, simultaneously burning fat while retaining and promoting lean muscle.

We will explore the use and principles behind using bodyweight with resistance, plyometric and isometric exercises, and how they are integrated into the rapid-workouts using various exercise systems. These systems include, but are not limited to, GPP (General Physical Preparedness) and Tabata timed-interval workouts, as well as repetition-based workouts. We will also explain how they impact on performance – taking 'your game' to the next level.

These workouts can be used as a standalone program but are

designed primarily for times when you can't make the gym, are away on holiday or business, strapped for time, or simply as booster 'add-ons' to your existing program. The workouts vary in difficulty, demarcated by a numbering system that enables you to select and employ them quickly.

Notes

[1] Significant level of fitness is quantified here as having trained for over a year and performed three or more sessions per week. Beginners are advised first to read *5 Minute Fitness* by Zen Martinoli, a detailed look at physical fitness, its science and introductory levels, the principles of which are echoed in this publication.

[2] 'Aerobic' means 'with oxygen' – when the body produces energy using oxygen in a complex and gradual process, breaking carbohydrates and fat down to produce energy. This sustainable production of energy is associated with continuous moderate exercise (CME), jogging, cycling and long-distance running, for example. We will explore how HIIT impacts on aerobic capacity.

[3] 'Anaerobic' means 'without oxygen'. This rapid-energy pathway is activated during short bursts of activity and is produced without the presence of oxygen, derived from the short supply of existing chemicals (phosphocreatine) in the body. Sprinting and weightlifting are good examples.

[4] 'Functional fitness' pertains to the combination of movements that relate to lifestyle or sports-specific movement. Functional exercises are compound movements that train a group of muscles simultaneously, as opposed to 'isolation exercises', which focus on a single muscle. Functional exercise does not only relate to day-to-day lifestyle movements (sitting, squatting, bending, etc.) but also specifically to sports. Training the muscles in an integrated fashion improves stability, co-ordination, agility, flexibility and balance, as well as increasing power, strength and speed.

Can short workouts be effective?

On a time-versus-results basis, they are potentially better.

Short workouts work by exploiting minimal time into maximum benefit using near-maximal or maximal exertion.In other words, we adopt a high-intensity approach and, in some instances, use HIIT – as with GPP and Tabata regimens, which are explained later in detail. Herein lies the key to success. The considerable physical exertion required in these rapid-workouts, by definition, means they have to be short, as the body can only sustain short bursts of high-intensity output before it needs to replenish its energy stores.

Despite this, the resulting training effects are extensive, unlocking the door to increased speed, power and strength – benefits not associated with longer, moderate CME. As well as improving anaerobic capacity, HIIT can also improve aerobic capacity, benefitting endurance as well as power athletes. HIIT is also viewed as the most time-efficient method of burning fat (see Tabata and GPP).

Although all the systems use bodyweight only, the individual workouts are characterised by time, tempo, rest, execution and level of difficulty to produce focused results in specific areas of fitness (speed, strength, power and endurance), as well as engendering improvements in stability, core strength, co-ordination, flexibility, motor skills and functional movement. Select the workouts that best complement your sporting/fitness goals.

They work best when applied to your existing program to enhance and boost your performance. Nevertheless, when planned correctly, they can provide a comprehensive standalone program, regarding which I have made recommendations and samples within the chapter on programs.

Important: I would, as a rule, always advocate the inclusion of CME components within your existing program, as these more gentle workouts give the body time to recover physically and neurologically, a welcome breather from the taxing demands of high-intensity training.

RAPID FITNESS EXERCISE METHODOLOGY

The next section outlines the protocols used with the rapid-workouts, their benefits and training goals. We explore the minutiae of the impact that various exercise stimuli have on us physiologically. We begin with the HIIT protocol and how it is exploited in terms of the workouts.

HIIT (High-Intensity Interval Training): characterised by high-intensity bursts followed by low-intensity or complete rest cycles.

HIIT circuits form the backbone of the rapid workouts featured in this book. This type of training is an ideal fit for the rapid workout, as we want to achieve maximum benefit in the limited time we have available. We will explore the origins and benefits behind HIIT training and the delivery systems of Tabata and GPP, also highlighting the pitfalls of high-intensity training and outlining good practice and application.

One may be excused for thinking that interval training is a recent exercise phenomenon due to its current popularity in the fitness industry. In fact, the Finnish Olympic long-distance runner Hannes Kolehmainen was using interval training in his workouts as early as 1912. Kolehmainen would perform five-to-ten repetitions of 1,000m in 3 minutes 5 seconds to improve his 10km-pace. Later, in the 1920s, Olympic champion Paavo Nurmi would integrate intervals of 6 x 400m into his long 10–20km runs to increase pace.

By the 1950s, interval training was being used by many athletes, including legends of the track Emil Zatopek and Roger Bannister;

the latter, of course, was the first to run a mile in under four minutes, combining both long and short intervals into his routine. As the popularity of interval training continued to grow among athletes, coaches and physiologists, so did the variety of ways the interval protocol could be manipulated, giving birth to HIIT, characterised by a burst-and-recover cycle. Peter Snell (800 and 1,500m Olympic champion) and his trainer in the 1960s developed an interval methodology of 10–15 seconds of very high-intensity sprints followed by 10–15 seconds of low-intensity jogging – what is now referred to as high-intensity interval training.

The intervening years and extensive investigative research on HIIT by exercise scientists has given rise to various permutations, the most notable (in my opinion) by Dr Izumi Tabatausing, a 20-second work/10-second rest regimen, explained later in greater detail.

The Benefits of Interval and High-Intensity Interval Training

In order to induce change, the principle of 'overload' comes into play. Placing the body under a variety of physical challenges constitutes an overload to the system, whereby physiological changes occur referred to as 'adaptations'. These in turn lead to increases in performance levels. We will go into the minutiae to discover the resultant adaptations and their impact on performance.

First, as previously mentioned in 5 Minute Fitness, we need to outline how the body produces energy and how this becomes relevant to the workouts in this volume.

Energy systems and ATP

ATP (adenosine triphosphate) is the energy molecule within a cell consisting of one part adenosine and three parts phosphate. One of the highly-charged phosphate strands breaks away, becoming

ADP (adenosine diphosphate). The molecule is then recycled and converted back to ATP to produce energy.

During aerobic exercise (moderate intensity), the aerobic energy system produces ATP in the presence of oxygen – a complex cycle that involves the gradual breakdown of glycogen (from carbohydrates) and fat (fatty acids), the result being a sustained manufacture of energy. This efficient energy-production process allows the exerciser to perform for long periods at a moderate pace, the balance of energy requirement versus energy production kept in equilibrium.

Anaerobic exercise (high and maximal intensity) requires an instant supply of ATP to support short, intense bursts of power output, created without the presence of oxygen. For short-burst maximal output (zero to ten seconds), ATP is derived from the limited supply of a high-energy compound called phosphocreatine already present within the muscles, referred to as the ATP-PC (anaerobic pathway). With its supply quickly depleted, the exerciser is forced to desist until the body has recycled further ATP. Working at a sub-maximal but high intensity (up to thirty seconds), energy is produced via the ATP-PC and lactic-acid system (anaerobic pathway) fuel, which at this point comes from both phosphocreatine and glycogen. As exercise time increases and intensity lowers, ATP is produced predominantly from the breakdown of glycogen until three minutes-plus, when anaerobic switches to aerobic and both glycogen and fatty acids are used to produce energy.

Both systems are employed to produce ATP to a greater or lesser degree, depending on the duration and intensity of exercise. These ratios will change in line with demand. For example, if while exercising at a moderate intensity you decide to gradually increase your pace, the ratio of energy pathways being used to produce ATP will shift – moving from aerobic to anaerobic. Continue to increase and you will eventually hit total failure; decrease and you will fall back into the more sustainable aerobic zone. The majority of sports will involve a combination of both systems working continuously to facilitate short bursts and sustained bouts of output. Understanding our body, how it produces energy and how this impacts on our performance and physiology are important factors in going forward.

Cardiovascular adaptations

The cardiovascular (derived from the Latin for heart and vessel) system comprises blood, heart and blood vessels. To improve the efficiency of the heart function in pumping blood to the working muscles, we engage in cardiovascular exercise normally associated with endurance training. Progressive increases in endurance training will activate adaptations whereby the heart muscle thickens and the left ventricle expands, improving heart function in terms of stroke volume (the volume of blood pumped per beat) and heart contractility (the forcefulness of each heart beat). As the heart grows stronger and is able to pump blood faster and with more force to the working muscles, so our performance levels increase. Similar cardiovascular adaptations occur with HIIT and, in some cases, can be superior to those occurring with endurance training.

Increasing VO2max:

VO2max (maximal oxygen consumption or, literally, V=volume, O2=oxygen, max=maximum) is measured as millilitres of oxygen used in one minute per kilogram of bodyweight (ml/kg/min). The measurement refers to the maximum amount of oxygen an individual is capable of utilising and converting into ATP during intense or maximal exercise.

For example, during aerobic exercise the demand for VO2

(oxygen consumption) increases in a linear relationship with exercise intensity. If an individual continues to increase their level of intensity until reaching their maximal level of exertion (i.e. absolute upper limit), this can be measured as their VO2max. This measurement is generally considered to be an accurate predictor of an individual's level of aerobic fitness – endurance athletes typically having a high VO2max. Research has intimated that HIIT is an essential training component for improving aerobic endurance.

A 1996 study by Dr Izumi Tabata and his team at the National Institute of Fitness and Sports in Tokyo yielded surprising results that challenged traditional assumptions about endurance training. Two controlled groups – one an endurance group, the other a high-intensity group – were prescribed specific training protocols. The purpose of the study was to improve the performance levels of the national Olympic cycling team – not only did the study prove highly effective at improving VO2max in the high-intensity group but it also generated a significant improvement of 28 per cent in their anaerobic capacity.

High Intensity Versus Endurance Training:			
Training Groups	Training Program	VO2max	Anaerobic Capacity
Endurance Training Group	Cycling at 70% VO2max for 60 minutes/daily. 5 days a week for 6 weeks.	Increase 10% (53 to 58 ml/kg/min)	No change
High-Intensity Training Group	Cycling at 170% VO2max. 8 x 20 sec sprints with 10 sec rest between. 5 days a week for 6 weeks.	Increase 14% (48 to 55 ml/kg/min)	Increased 28%

Data from 'Effect of moderate-intensity endurance and high-intensity intermittent training on anaerobic capacity and VO2max' by I. Tabata et al (1996), *Medicine & Science in Sports & Exercise*, 28(10): 1327–1330.

Another study (much of which followed the original) was undertaken by Daussin et al. (2008), which had men and women participating over eight weeks in both HIIT and CME programs. HIIT participants came out on top, showing improvements of 15 per cent in VO2max compared to 9 per cent improvement in the endurance trial – reinforcing the idea that HIIT can contribute to making the body more efficient at producing energy and, in turn, improve your cardio-respiratory fitness, enabling the individual to perform faster for longer.

Increasing mitochondria

Mitochondria are the powerhouses of skeletal muscle (muscles attached to bone) cells and are responsible for manufacturing ATP. They work like a digestive system, absorbing then breaking down nutrients to convert into energy for the cell. An increase in the density (size and number) of mitochondria allows you to produce more energy for longer. For many years the increasing of mitochondrial density, or 'mitochondrial biogenesis', was thought to occur only from extreme endurance training (when mitochondria use oxygen to break down fat and carbohydrates for energy/ATP). However, it is now recognised as a hallmark adaptation of HIIT (Gibala, 2009). Research shows that the increase in oxidative enzymes (proteins in mitochondria that quicken the rate at which ATP is produced) created during endurance exercise can be equalled and, in some cases, bettered with HIIT. The complex molecular pathways that lead to mitochondrial density are still being explored. However, it appears that HIIT achieves similar results using different signalling pathways. One knock-on effect of increased mitochondrial density is a raised anaerobic threshold.

Increasing anaerobic threshold

'Anaerobic threshold' (AT) refers to the point at which lactic acid (waste product) begins to accumulate in the bloodstream, bringing exercise to a stop.

Increasing your anaerobic threshold enables the working muscles to work harder for longer, becoming more efficient at withstanding and removing their waste products. As your anaerobic capacity improves (Tabata, 1996), so do does your ability to raise your AT (also predetermined to a certain extent by genetics), enabling you to sustain a higher intensity for longer.

Referring back to ATP, we now understand how it's produced and for what type of mechanical work. During anaerobic exercise we reach our AT rapidly, as ATP stores deplete and lactic acid builds, reaching the point where the production of lactate (produced by the anaerobic system) is higher than its removal. During aerobic exercise the ratio of anaerobic-aerobic is low enough for generated lactate to be easily removed, while the aerobic pathway continues to create ATP to sustain a comfortable intensity. It is only when the speed/intensity is increased that this ratio changes until, eventually, the body again cannot remove lactate quickly enough to sustain performance.

Using HIIT and training our body close to its anaerobic limit, we improve our ability to remove lactate more effectively, pushing back the anaerobic threshold. AT will vary from person to person and from sport to sport. Untrained individuals typically have a low AT (approximately 55 per cent of VO2max), highly trained athletes a high AT (approximately 80–90 per cent of VO2max), as illustrated below. See Fig.2 (p.13) to view AT in relation to an RPE (Rate of Perceived Exertion) chart.

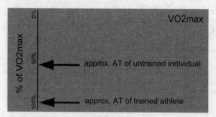

Burning more fat and understanding EPOC

It has long been considered that the ideal 'training zone' for burning fat is during aerobic exercise at between 60–70 per cent of your maximum effort – alternatively, 60–70 per cent of your MHR (maximum heart rate)[1] if using a heart-rate monitor. This is, indeed, a productive training zone but requires considerable time invested. Let's take a look at how working at high intensity for considerably less time can engender better results for fat burning.

For the purposes of this book, we will use an intensity numbering system called an RPE Scale.[2] RPE allows us to self-evaluate our level of intensity without any equipment. The system requires an accurate appraisal of how hard you are working and is specific to your current fitness level. Numbers 3–7 approximately correlate to 50–90 per cent of MHR, 7–10 to approximately 90–100 per cent of MHR.

So numbers 3–4 would constitute a sustainable aerobic fat-burning level; 4–5 moves into aerobic endurance; 6–7 into the high-intensity, less sustainable anaerobic; and 8–10 into short-burst, extremely high-intensity moving into ultra-high intensity (VO2max). Going forward, we will use this scale to illustrate where the specific workouts sit within the RPE Scale. Fig.1 shows an RPE chart with the workout zones superimposed to give you a clearer idea. Fig.2 is an earlier graphic highlighting where the approximate AT of trained and untrained individuals shows within VO2max.

Fig. 1 RPE Chart

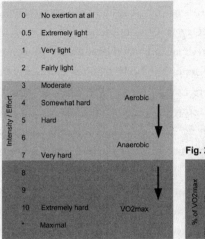

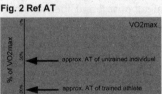

Fig. 2 Ref AT

Guide RPE:

3. Moderate – easy to perform.

4. Somewhat hard – fairly easy.

5. Hard – breathing and working a little hard.

6. Harder – beginning to breathe heavily.

7. Very hard – very challenging, breathing very hard.

8. Working and breathing seriously hard.

9. Approaching upper limits, working and breathing at near-maximal limits.

10. Extremely hard – working and breathing at maximal intensity.

On the surface, it is logical that aerobic exercise has long been considered the best route to burn fat when energy is derived from the breakdown of fatty acids and glycogen (carbohydrates) in a sustainable, continuous process. However, it has been suggested that more fat can be metabolised as a result of high-intensity exercise with

80–100 per cent of maximum effort, or between 6 and 10 on the RPE Scale. This has to do with a metabolic post-exercise process called EPOC (Excess Post-Exercise Oxygen Consumption).

EPOC occurs after both aerobic and anaerobic exercise, restoring the body to its pre-exercise state. The body requires more oxygen post-exercise than it did pre-exercise to re-oxygenate the blood, replenish energy stores and restore body temperature, heart-rate and breathing to pre-exercise levels. This post-exercise work increases metabolism[3] and fuel consumption – hence burning additional fat to assist the process. Research (Bahr and Sejersted, 1987, *Journal of Applied Physiology*) shows that EPOC consumption increases in line with the level of exercise intensity. In addition, the higher the intensity, the longer EPOC works – in some cases up to twenty-four hours post-exercise.

Put into simpler terms, the harder you work, the harder your body has to work post-exercise to return itself to its pre-exercise state, burning more calories/fat for longer. Viewed on a time-versus-results basis, HIIT is more time-efficient proposition for burning fat.

To illustrate this further, Dr Trembley (Physical Activity Sciences Laboratory, Laval University, Canada) concluded that it is possible to burn up to nine times more fat with HIIT compared to endurance exercise. For the study, one group entered into a 20-week endurance training (ET) program, the other a 15-week HIIT program. The ET group expended twice the energy of the HIIT group yet, despite this, the HIIT group had a higher reduction in subcutaneous adiposity (subcutaneous fat).[4] When the figures were adjusted for the respective energy cost of training, the results proved remarkable. The results showed that the decrease in the sum of six skin-fold measurements (body-fat measurements taken from bicep, triceps, calf, back, hips and abdomen) induced by the HIIT program was nine times greater than that induced by the ET program.

Notes

[1] MHR being how fast your heart can contract in one minute. There are many formulae available to calculate MHR, the age-adjusted being the most common (available from the Internet, you will also require a heart monitor when exercising).

[2] 'Perceived Exertion as an Indicator of Somatic Stress', G. Borg (1970), *Scandinavian Journal of Rehabilitation Medicine*, 2(2), 92–98.

[3] Metabolism refers to the biochemical processes that occur within the body to maintain life. These processes allow us to reproduce, grow, repair damage and respond to our environment.

[4] Subcutaneous fat is situated directly under the skin. It is measured with a skin-fold calliper to estimate total body fat.

Promote muscle gains while burning fat

Increasing our metabolic rate with HIIT and resistance training increases the production of anabolic[1] hormone testosterone and human-growth hormone HRH (*Journal of Strength and Conditioning*), stimulating muscle mass and burning fat.

This increased level of anabolic hormones contributes to the growth and mineralisation of bone as well as muscle mass (hypertrophy). In contrast, excessive endurance training has the opposite catabolic[2] effect on the body, producing the hormone cortisol, breaking muscle down to use as energy.

So as well as being ultra-efficient at burning fat, high-intensity exercise not only retains hard-earned muscle but also stimulates growth. HIIT sets off an increase in thin and thick myofilaments (protein cords within a muscle fibre), resulting in size and strength adaptations. One only needs to look at body types attributed to different sports to observe the impact exercise protocols have on muscular composition. Sprinters, for example, have powerful, muscular frames capable of generating short bursts of incredible speed and power. Long-distance runners, their bodies having adapted to this requirement, exhibit the exact opposite, the product of extreme endurance training – sinewy, light and economic.

Notes

[1] Anabolism is, effectively, the constructive metabolism. This sequence of chemical processes constructs complex molecules (polymers) from simple small molecules (monomers), allowing the body to make new cells while maintaining all the tissues. The analogy would be the bricks of a house being monomers and the house itself a polymer. This translates to simple molecules called amino acids (monomers) going through a series of anabolic chemical reactions, building into larger, more complex proteins (polymers). These anabolic reactions manufacture a range of finished products, including the growth of bone and muscle mass. Typical anabolic hormones would be HRH, testosterone and oestrogen in women.

[2] Catabolism is the reverse of anabolism, breaking polymers into monomers and releasing energy in the process. The energy is used on a cellular level up to entire body movements. This deconstruction process occurs when we eat food, the organic material being stored inside the molecules of ATP (as referenced earlier). The newly-created store of energy is then used to fuel anabolic reactions. When catabolism produces more energy than anabolism requires, the excess energy is stored as fat or glycogen. The opposite occurs on occasions such as excessive endurance exercise. In this instance, once catabolism has used fat and glycogen stores, it will revert to protein as fuel, thus breaking muscle down to fuel the anabolic processes. Typical catabolic hormones would be cortisol, glucagon and adrenalin.

Developing fast-twitch muscle

We investigate later how training explosively develops our speed, power and strength – specifically our fast-twitch muscle fibres. Our bodies contain three types of skeletal muscle responsible for generating varying degrees of force: Type 1, Type 2a and Type 2x. These are general classifications, as modern techniques in fibre typing indicate that fibre types exist on a continuum consisting of multiple variants. For clarity and simplicity, we will stay with the general types.

Type 1 fibres: referred to as slow-twitch fibres, slow-contraction velocity fibres – or slow oxidative (SO) fibres – are suited to endurance training. They are red in colour due to large volumes of myoglobin (protein containing oxygen) and contain high amounts of mitochondria and capillaries. Their capacity to generate large amounts of ATP via the aerobic metabolism makes them highly resistant to fatigue and able to sustain repeated low-level contractions.

Type 2a fibres: these are also known as intermediate fast-twitch fibres and are pinkish-red in colour, as they contain high amounts of myoglobin and mitochondria (although not quite as much as Type 1). They are viewed as a combination of both Type 1 and Type 2 and thus produce ATP, via both the aerobic and anaerobic metabolisms, at a rapid rate. This hybrid production process also lends them the name fast oxidative/glycolytic fibres. They contract five times faster than Type 1 fibres and are highly resistant to fatigue, although not as efficient as Type 1.

Type 2x fibres: these fast-twitch fibres are also known as fast glycolytic fibres. They are white in colour, as they contain low levels of myoglobin and mitochondria. ATP is manufactured via the anaerobic metabolism and derived from the instant supply of glycogen already present in the muscle. These fibres contract extremely rapidly – ten times faster than Type 1 – but fatigue quickly.

By focusing on these 'higher threshold' fibres using speed-, strength-

Fibre Type	Type 1	Type 2a	Type 2x
Intensity Used	Moderate	High	Maximal
Contraction Speed (Milliseconds)	Slow 90-140 ms	Fast 50-100 ms	Very Fast 40-90 ms
Contraction Force	Low	High	Very High
Resistance to Fatigue	High	Intermediate	Low
Myoglobin Content	High	High	Low
Glycogen Content	Low	High	High
Mitochondrial Density	High	High	Low
Capillary Density	High	Intermediate	Low
Oxidative Capacity	High	Intermediate	Low
Motor Neuron Size	Small	Large	Very Large

and power-dominant activities, we encourage our nervous system and fibres to behave in a fast-twitch manner. Using plyometrics (activities that enable a muscle to reach maximum force) and resistance training (bodyweight resistance, for this book) both alone and combined (known as complex training), we can develop the ability to recruit high numbers of fast-twitch fibres neurologically, via signals from the brain to motor units prompting rapid activation, as well as increasing their size and strength. We will investigate later in this book the combination of speed and strength training to improve 'rate of force' (the time it takes to produce maximal force during exercise) or, more simply, *power*.

It is important to note that we are born with our own genetic blueprint of slow- and fast-twitch fibres, the average person comprising approximately 50 per cent fast-twitch and 50 per cent slow-twitch. This proportion, however, can differ from person to person, lending the individual more of a propensity to excel at a given sport; long-distance runners will have a higher ratio of slow to fast-twitch fibres, sprinters a higher ratio of fast to slow-twitch fibres. Although the quantities of fibres are predetermined, we can, with training, transform their characteristics. Although the exact mechanism for fibre conversion is unclear, the suggestion is that it is neuromuscular.

It is possible we could have as much as 40 per cent control over our muscle-fibre type (Dr J. Simoneau and Dr C. Bouchard). Alternative research has this figure lower, at a more modest 10 per cent, the rest being predetermined by genetics. Whatever the exact percentage, it is universally recognised within research literature that inter-conversions between Types 2a and 2x are possible with training. However, there is still considerable disagreement over the capacity for Types 1 and 2 to inter-convert. The *Journal of Strength and Conditioning* published an article whereby they were categorical that one cannot inter-convert between fibre types 1 and 2 and that change could only occur within sub-types (i.e. within slow or fast variant sub-types). It is also unclear which muscle types (i.e. bicep, hamstring, etc.) are more susceptible to change than others. Research remains ongoing.

What we do know for definite is that we can modify, with explosive and resistance activity, Type 2a fibres into Type 2x fibres and vice versa, creating more responsive, stronger and powerful bodies. Conversely, it is logical to assume that we could 'detrain' our explosive potential by solely engaging in activities that typically use Type 1 fibres. So to remain predominantly fast-twitch-centric, we would avoid including too much slow-twitch activity within our program – too much roadwork, for example, although good for the aerobic engine, would not benefit the explosive power requirements of, for example, a boxer. The correct ratio here would be chiefly high-intensity sessions: pads, bags, speedball, sprints and sparring interspersed (sparingly) with low-intensity roadwork and low-intensity skipping, etc. There are many permutations with the above example but the idea is to be sport-specific – although factoring in *other activities* is vital for our all-round fitness and injury prevention (see Chapter 6).

Exercise adherence

As well as the multitude of physiological benefits, there are practical and psychological advantages of adding HIIT routines to your program. Time efficiency, variety and equal or improved results in less time all contribute to a greater likelihood of adhering to an exercise program. Nevertheless, there are considerations.

A cautionary word

We have explored the many benefits of engaging in high-intensity exercise, of which there are many. However, it is important to highlight the pitfalls and employ a sensible, balanced approach. You must initially have a sufficient platform of aerobic fitness before you attempt this type of intensity. The cardiovascular system needs to be conditioned, as do the muscles, to cope with the output required; literally jumping straight in could be significantly harmful to your health. A common mistake among the untrained is to view HIIT routines as the shortcut alternative to traditional endurance training. The 'time-efficient strategy' to make fast gains is an attitude indicative of our quick-fix culture and potentially detrimental to your health. To reiterate: cultivate a base aerobic fitness; build towards a safe and conditioned platform; and then enjoy the gains of HIIT.

HIIT is not the panacea of all aerobic conditioning; we are designed to perform endurance activities as well as sprinting, lifting and jumping. Conditioning your body aerobically with moderate training, as well as anaerobically, is the key to success, longevity and rounded fitness.

When you are ready to introduce HIIT workouts to your program, you should do so with adequate breaks and recovery time. Excessive use can engender dramatic increases in the catabolic hormones cortisol and epinephrine, leading to muscle wastage and injuries. In addition, training too frequently at a high intensity can lower testosterone levels in men and progesterone levels in women, as well as depleting HRH levels instead of encouraging growth. To avoid this and capitalise on the benefits, use a common-sense approach.

Recommended use: three times per week. Cycle weeks on or off, depending on your program. A practical approach is four weeks on and four weeks off. Recovery time of 48 hours between workouts is a sensible anaerobic guideline. The volume of workouts that any one individual can perform will be dependent on their health, aerobic capacity and general lifestyle. If you are not sleeping well, eating badly and stressed, you are already compromised hormonally. Adding further stress with HIIT and producing more cortisol would only lead to injury and health issues down the line. Adequate sleep and diet, coupled with good health and aerobic conditioning, is the ideal starting point.

TABATA – ULTRA-HIGH INTERVAL TRAINING: THE DETAILS

Let us now examine the different regimen used to deliver high-intensity exercise with the rapid workouts. First is Tabata, the benefits of which we have already covered. As alluded to previously, Tabata is a 2:1 ratio of work to rest, consisting of eight cycles of 20-second ultra-high intensity intervals interspersed with 10-second rests. To be more precise, all-out effort at 170 per cent of your VO2max is the criterion. Using our REP chart, 'maximal' would signify where you need to be in terms of intensity. To enjoy the full benefits of Tabata, it is a prerequisite to execute each interval 'all-out' – there are no half-measures, as brutal as it may feel. When performed correctly, the final rounds feel almost impossible to execute. However, it is important to note that one can still benefit from Tabata by working at a submaximal intensity and work towards the maximal over a period of time. These are by far the most taxing of all HIIT regimens, so approach with care and caution.

To achieve the required level of intensity, we need to employ specific bodyweight exercises that are challenging enough to exploit the minimal workout time of twenty seconds – yet not too intense that we cannot complete the entire workout (eight cycles of twenty seconds). Example: eight cycles of press-ups for most individuals is too demanding to complete, let alone perform consistently at a high level, whereas eight cycles of crunches may be insufficiently taxing to achieve the required high intensity for the protocol (of course, there are exceptions to the rule). The exercises designated for Tabata in this book are selected to represent a generic challenge to anyone with a regular exercise regime or any sportsperson, with an emphasis on intensity determined by the volume of work (amount of repetitions) completed per 20-second cycle. Seasoned exercisers may consider substituting some exercises with more advanced propositions (e.g. squat jumps to replace standard squats). It will become quickly evident once these workouts are performed which are most suited to your current ability.

Borg CR10 Scale

Intensity / Effort		
0	No exertion at all	
0.5	Extremely light	
1	Very light	
2	Fairly light	
3	Moderate	
4	Somewhat hard	
5	Hard	
6		
7	Very hard	
8		
9		
10	Extremely hard	
*	Maximal	Tabata Zone

GPP intervals

The term 'General Physical Preparedness' originates from a Russian system of coaching designed to target general areas of fitness in the preparatory phase prior to an athlete's SPP (Specific Physical Preparedness) or sport-specific training phase. The purpose of GPP is to create a broad foundation of fitness that can be applied to a wide range of tasks, including those pertaining to an athlete's chosen sport. This all-round-fitness protocol is intended to provide balanced physical conditioning to the broadest range of demands, including speed, strength, endurance, functionality and flexibility, using all major muscle groups and joints. Adding this component to your training fills in the gaps, or areas that specific training might neglect, thereby not only creating a base level of fitness but also protecting against injury through imbalances. An example might be a power-lifter who, when training with GPP, would avoid maximal-strength work and instead concentrate on sprinting training, rowing or other non-related activities.

This component of training can benefit either the regular exerciser or sportsperson who is in a prepatory phase or, used sparingly, between SPP sessions. GPP routines feature throughout the book and fit nicely into what we are trying to achieve with short, effective, convenient workouts. The GPP workouts will combine plyometric and resistance exercises, featuring both as timed high-intensity intervals and repetition-based bodyweight circuits. Other mini-workouts will focus with more specificity on speed, power or strength alone.

GPP high-intensity intervals

Although not 'ultra-high', GPP intervals will engender all the benefits generally associated with high-intensity interval training. The book will offer a variety of ratios of work to rest: for example, three minutes' work to one minute's rest (3:1). In this case, the exerciser would work for three minutes in thirty-second continuous blocks, resting for a full minute before starting a further circuit for a prescribed number of circuits. Another permutation might be a 2:1 ratio – forty seconds of high intensity to twenty seconds of moderate intensity (or active rest) for three minutes non-stop. To give you a guide to the work intensity of any given GPP interval, aim between 6 and 7

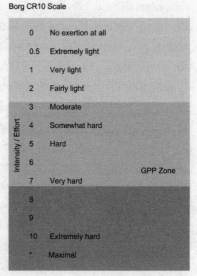

Borg CR10 Scale

0	No exertion at all
0.5	Extremely light
1	Very light
2	Fairly light
3	Moderate
4	Somewhat hard
5	Hard
6	
7	Very hard
8	
9	
10	Extremely hard
*	Maximal

Intensity / Effort

GPP Zone

on the RPE chart. Complete rest is obviously 0 (no exertion at all); 'active rest' would be between 2 and 3 (fairly light to moderate).

Resistance, plyometric, isometric and complex training exercises

Having outlined Tabata and GPP intervals, we can now look at the different types of exercises that constitute these workouts. In addition, there will also be workouts independent of HIIT circuits that will concentrate and isolate specific components of fitness, strength, speed or power. Let's start by looking at resistance training (you may already have a handle on the principles here – however, the point is to outline the relevance to bodyweight exercises).

Essentially, any exercises involving the lengthening of a muscle (eccentric) and shortening of a muscle (concentric) are referred to as 'isotonic'. Conversely, isometric contraction involves no change in muscle length and is static in comparison. Now let's look at the different forms of isotonic and isometric training, and how they combine.

Resistance training is overloading a muscle group to engender adaptations in strength, endurance or growth (hypertrophy). Through a combination of repetitions, sets, tempo and exercises, these specific gains can be manifested. The benefits are manifold and include increases in muscle size, bone density, joint function, ligament and tendon strength (particularly with isometric resistance, explained later on), metabolism, heart function and, of course, associated cosmetic benefits! Before looking at how resistance applies to bodyweight, to best understand the principles it is simpler to visualise using an external load/resistance.

Typically, to target absolute or maximal strength, one would perform between one to five reps using a heavy load (80–90 per cent of your 1RM)[1] executed with maximum force and significant rest between sets of two to five minutes. To target hypertrophy (growth) and strength, one would perform six to twelve reps using a load between 60–80 per cent of your 1RM with a slower contraction, resting for ninety seconds to two minutes between sets. Endurance would see you perform 13–25 reps at 40–60 per cent of your 1RM, again with a slower contraction but with even shorter rests between sets of 30–90 seconds. These ranges are not set in stone (one could be training hypertrophy between 12–15, for example, somewhere near the crossover). In addition, if we wanted to improve *power* with an external load, we would use a resistance representing 50–60 per cent of our 1RM but execute the lift-fast contraction for four to six reps.

How does this translate to bodyweight? It is important to note that *Rapid Fitness* is not a bodybuilding bible; if your aim is to build huge muscles or attain boundless strength gains, there are equipment-based books out there to help you on your way. Nevertheless, bodyweight does present, to most people, a considerable resistance and can engender noteworthy gains in muscular strength, growth and endurance. By modifying exercise difficulty, intensity and tempo, we can reproduce similar benefits. Prescribing reps in terms of *bodyweight* represents a different challenge from one individual to another.

An example would be prescribing 10–12 reps of a standard press-up to three people of various strengths: the weakest may able to perform only six reps and this would constitute strength training; the next may perform the required range of 10–12 reps (strength and growth); the third may be capable of twenty reps, which moves him into the endurance end of the strength continuum. To achieve a similar training effect of strength and growth in all three, the first could perform an easier, modified press-up for 10–12 reps, the second could remain the same and the third perform a more difficult variable press-up, or perform the existing press-up at a slower tempo for 10–12 reps. We can, with adjustment, modification and application, achieve good results but there *are* limits with strength and growth using bodyweight only and, eventually, there will be a ceiling to further gains. At this point, external load is required.

The resistance rapid workouts will be prescribed within the eight-to-twenty-rep range to cover strength, growth and endurance in a total-body approach. High-end strength one-to-five reps are omitted as, in general, the majority of bodyweight exercises can be performed for more than five reps. However, this excludes isometric-strength training, which will be explained later.

What about power (speed strength)? We can develop power by dynamically shifting our bodyweight using plyometric and (static) isometric exercise. We will also look at how the combination of the two (complex training) can lead to even greater improvements in power.

Note

[1] 1RM indicates the maximum weight one can push for one repetition only.

CHAPTER TWO

PLYOMETRIC TRAINING

Plyometric exercises are maximal muscular contractions aimed at improving an individual's power and explosive reactions. Characterised as jumping, hopping and bounding, plyometrics were first used by East German athletic coaches in the 1970s. Since then, these 'dynamic-resistance' exercises have become commonplace with professional and amateur athletes. The training aim is to enable a muscle to reach maximum strength in as short a time as possible – referred to as 'speed strength' but more commonly as 'power'.

Before we investigate plyometric exercise, let us clarify speed strength: it is the ability of the neuromuscular system[1] to produce the greatest possible impulse in the shortest possible time. There are three components to speed strength: 'starting strength', 'explosive strength' and 'reactive strength'.

Starting strength is the force created at the beginning of a movement; it is the ability to recruit or 'fire' as many motor units as possible instantaneously. Explosive strength is the ability to continue this initiated force as fast as possible. This time is quantified as the rate of force (the time it takes to produce maximum force during a movement). Reactive strength, or a 'stretch-shortening' cycle, is the creation and usage of kinetic energy during movement, explained in detail later.

At this point, it is important to understand that being strong does not necessarily translate to explosive strength. 'The ability to produce maximal forces in minimal time is called explosive strength. Strong people do not necessarily possess explosive strength.' (Dr Vladimir Zatsiorsky, 1995)

Developing explosive strength is generally associated with moving heavy loads at speed or, to be more precise: 'Exercises used to develop explosive strength are defined as those in which the initial rate of concentric force production is maximal or near maximal and is maintained throughout range of motion of the exercise.'[2] Although this generally refers to executing an external heavy load at speed (e.g. power-lifting), we can create a high-force production with bodyweight exercises using multiple jumps, bounds and depth jumps, all of which will significantly contribute to your explosive strength. In addition, starting strength, explosive strength and overall speed strength can be meaningfully improved *without moving* by using isometrics (explained later in terms of overcoming isometrics).

Coming back to plyometric exercises, these exercises are centred on a muscle rapidly stretching (in doing so, creating a type of kinetic 'elastic energy') and then rapidly shortening (releasing the kinetic energy) to engender maximum speed and power in the shortest possible time, referred to as the 'stretch-shortening cycle' (SSC) or 'reactive strength'.

The emphasis here is on rapid contraction, exploding from the eccentric phase into the concentric phase; the faster the time, the greater the force created, hence training will increase speed strength/power. These types of exercises are used in virtually all the rapid-workouts and are expressed in various degrees of difficulty/intensity, depending on the focus and aim of the individual workout. The emphasis with plyometric exercise is always on quality, not quantity.

There will be workouts designed to improve specific abilities for vertical, horizontal, lateral and directional power. Some may be more specific to your requirements, although *all* will benefit your complete performance.

Important note: in addition to the general safety advice at the beginning of the first chapter, ensure you are well conditioned with good leg strength before attempting 'plyos'. Start with smaller jumps and build up. Aim to land softly with good landing technique. Exercise-execution guidelines will be provided per exercise within the exercise portfolio.

Notes:

[1] The combination of nervous system and muscles working together to permit movement is known as the neuromuscular system.

[2] Stone, M.H. (1993). 'Position Statement. Literature review: Explosive Exercises and Training' *NSCA Journal*, 15(3): 7–14.

CHAPTER THREE

ISOMETRIC TRAINING

M uscle activation can be defined as three phases: concentric (shortening of a muscle), isometric (no change in length) and eccentric (lengthening of a muscle). These three phases are termed triphasic. So in every dynamic movement, there is an isometric component.

Isometric-resistance exercises are performed from a static position involving no 'range of motion' (ROM). The joint angle and muscle length remain the same during isometric contraction, in contrast to the dynamic muscle lengthening and shortening phases of a movement. Strength gains are considered to be only at the angle of the joint, although some argue that benefits fan out for up to 15° either side of the joint angle. Let's look at the origins and go into further detail.

Famous 'strongman' Alexander Zass was a great advocate of isometric training. When incarcerated during the Second World War, he would push and pull on the chains and bars of his cell. As his strength exponentially increased, he was able to eventually break free with his bare hands. In later years he went on to catalogue and market his ideas.

Isometric exercises have been used since time immemorial and form the basis of many yoga and Pilates static 'holds'. In recent times their independent use has become less common in mainstream fitness, as they present a less attractive or interesting proposition compared to the multitude of alternatives, coupled with the fact that they have no commercial value in terms of equipment. Detractors will also allude to drawbacks such as central nervous system (CNS) fatigue, decreased speed, reduced co-ordination and reduced muscle elasticity and yes, this may be the case if overused, but, when used sparingly and properly sequenced with appropriate rest, they present an extra dimension in strength, ligament and tendon building, as well as increased ability in motor-unit recruitment and improved speed of movement.

THE TWO FORMS OF ISOMETRIC CONTRACTIONS: 'YIELDING ISO-METRIC' AND 'OVERCOMING ISOMETRIC'

Yielding isometric is where either a weight or bodyweight is lowered and then held at a predetermined joint angle for a predetermined amount of time. An example would be lowering from a press-up start position into mid-range, then holding for a pre-determined time, such as 20–40 seconds. This type of isometric is perceived to be more effective for acute-strength short-term gains and muscle hypertrophy. In addition, this type of 'iso' is used to develop better deceleration (ability to stop quickly and stabilise) in athletes.

A further use for yielding isometrics is to hold for maximum time to work on ROM using EQI (eccentric quasi-isometric) principles.

EQI explained: this is when a yielding isometric is held mid-range (also referred to as the 'bottom' of a movement). This is held for maximum time; as you fatigue, you sink a little lower (the eccentric phase) and, in doing so, gradually increase your mobility (ROM). Pulling deeper into the stretch adds more stability and flexibility to the end ranges of mobility and reduces the risk of injury going forward. Use EQIs to elicit great strength and mobility benefits.

Overcoming isometric is where the joint and muscle work against an immovable force, like pressing against a wall or pulling against a fixed object– these are typically six-to-ten-second maximal contractions (but can be as low as three seconds). This type of isometric training is considered superior to yielding isometrics for long-term strength development. Over time these repeated maximal force contractions against an immovable object result in considerable strength adaptations and elevated motor-unit recruitment. This type of 'iso' is used to develop better acceleration (the ability to speed up quickly) in athletes.

When using isometric exercises, it's important to define our objectives:

To improve your explosive strength (a component of speed strength, as previously mentioned), overcoming isometric exercises would be more beneficial. 'Explosive strength is developed with tension increased with maximum speed.' (Verkhoshansky, 1977)

To develop muscle gains (and strength), yielding isometrics would be more appropriate. Hypertrophy (muscle gain) is developed with longer 30–60-second sequences. 'It is thought that the longer muscle contraction leads to blood flow occlusion, increasing metabolite concentrations.' (Kraemer and Fleck, 2004)

How can a static contraction improve speed strength?

To best understand this question, we need to look at how motor units work.

Muscle fibres are grouped together into *motor units* served by one nerve that delivers a signal to the muscle fibres (neuromuscular system). The motor units of slow-twitch fibres usually contain no more than 300 fibres, whereas the motor units of fast-twitch fibres are not only larger but contain more fibres, ranging from hundreds to thousands.

On receiving a signal, all muscle fibres within a motor unit contract. The units which fire will be dependent on the level of *force* required. When the requirement is minimal, it is the smaller motor nerves requiring the least amount of stimulation which excite their motor units to contract first – slow-twitch muscle fibres have the smallest nerves, and so will perform easy-to-moderate effort. Once the neural drive exceeds moderate, the larger motor nerves belonging to fast-twitch Type 2a fibres will be stimulated into action to assist its slow-twitch counterparts. The greatest amount of excitation is required to stimulate the largest motor nerves of Type 2x fibres, recruited only when effort reaches near-maximal.

To summarise: slow-twitch motor units contract the slowest and with least force, activated by the least stimulus; fast-twitch motor units contract much faster and with greater force but require considerable neural drive to activate. When considering an isometric contraction (particularly in overcoming isometric), the greatest possible amount of motor units are fired during these highly-intense maximal contractions, making these exercises particularly effective at training motor-unit recruitment. It is important to note that fibre recruitment is accumulative, not *either/or* – meaning that fast-twitch fibres do not fire instead of slow-twitch, they fire *as well as*; each fibre type assists its precursor until all fire simultaneously during a maximal contraction.

With this in mind, we can now understand how speed strength is improved by developing the rate of force dynamically (with plyometrics) but also, in this case, statically (isometric). The previous paragraph tells us that muscle-fibre recruitment is directly related to the force or power required to accomplish a movement, not the speed needed to perform it. For example, one can pedal a bicycle on a (low-intensity) high gear *quickly*, which requires minimal force – in this instance, slow-twitch muscle fibres would be facilitating a *fast movement*. Conversely, one could stimulate fast-twitch fibres into action by lifting a heavy weight with a *slow movement* requiring maximal force.

In most sports, however, an increase in effort will translate to an increase in speed. A sprinter or swimmer, for example, when increasing effort will usually increase speed, which is why speed and power are commonly mentioned together. But what the aforementioned analogies show is that fast-twitch motor units can be trained without movement, meaning speed strength/power can be improved with isometric training. It is the intent to move quickly which is important, whether the action is dynamic or static, therefore the explosive tension created during an isometric contraction is conducive to speed development.

When approaching an isometric contraction, keep full body contraction in mind. Initially, this will feel counter-intuitive, as we are conditioned to 'firing' the motor units of the agonist muscles (muscles that contract during a movement – i.e. prime mover being the pectorals during a press-up) during a contraction and not the antagonists (opposing muscle – i.e. back during a press-up) at the same time. With this in mind, focus on full-body firing, tensing *every* muscle during contraction.

Important note: if you suffer from high blood pressure or a heart condition, it is inadvisable to perform isometric exercises.

Combine strength and plyometric work with *complex training*.

CHAPTER FOUR

COMPLEX TRAINING

Research has suggested that the most potent method for increasing power is combining strength and speed exercises, referred to as complex training. In doing so, we increase the 'rate of force'(the time it takes to produce maximum force during a movement).

In addition, Verkhoshansky (1977) concluded that the combination of both static and dynamic exercises – for example, a (static) isometric squat hold followed by a (dynamic) squat jump – was potentially 20 per cent better at developing speed strength than dynamic exercise alone. So the combination of strength exercises, either isotonic or isometric, coupled with plyometric exercises can lead to significant gains in speed strength.

This training is based on an initial isometric resistance exercise preparing the CNS (central nervous system) and activating the Type 2x fibres (responsible for explosive movement), making them available for the ensuing dynamic plyometric exercise and resulting in greater 'rate of force'.

If you are an athlete, this type of training is suitable during any phase but, as with all exercise that hits your CNS hard, needs to be used sparingly and properly cycled.

CHAPTER FIVE

CORE EXERCISE

The muscles of the core reside in the central area of the body (the trunk) and are instrumental in all functional movements. Misquoted and misunderstood, the word 'core' is often used interchangeably with abs. The *rectus abdominis*, more commonly known as 'abs' or 'six pack', has one specific, limited function and that is to flex the spine (forward bend). The muscles of the core, however, are comprised of many different muscles playing various roles in stabilising the spine and pelvis and, in doing so, facilitate the generation and transfer of power to the extremities (limbs). The core is the centre of extremity function.

When training the core, it is important to understand that the trunk itself comprises inner and outer units. Inner units are responsible for stabilising while outer units initiate movement, working together in symbiosis. Synergy between both is vital to produce stability of the spine for the ensuing movement; neglecting inner-unit development can lead to complications and injury, inhibiting potential gains in speed and power. Below are the generally accepted main core muscles – note that some outer units also provide stabilisation.

The main player in terms of the inner units is the transverse abdominis (TrA), which is utilised during all movements and engages the pelvic floor and diaphragm in conjunction with the obliques when drawing the navel into the spine – a technique that must be executed correctly to be effective. To perform this action correctly, as your stomach hollows try and visualise touching your spine with your navel. It is important you breathe during contraction. Train the slow-twitch inner units first, as they fatigue less quickly than their fast-twitch outer-unit counterparts. This also reflects the natural sequencing of engagement.

The stabilising inner units are: transverse abdominis, multifidus, pelvic floor, diaphragm and fibres at the back of the internal oblique.

The movement-initiating outer units are: rectus abdominis, external and internal obliques, erector spinae.

Transverse abdominis: these are the deepest of the core muscles and lie under the obliques, acting as a girdle to compress and stabilise the trunk and support the abdominal viscera (the internal organs enclosed within the abdominal cavity).

Rectus abdominis: this is the long muscle referred to as the 'six pack' that extends across the front of the abdomen and is used to flex the trunk.

External obliques: these are situated around the waist on the side and front of the abdomen. They stabilise and rotate the trunk and provide some lateral flexion (side bend).

Internal obliques: these lie under the external obliques and run in the opposite direction. They are the main stabilisers of the trunk and provide lateral flexion.

Erector spinae: these run from the neck to the lower back and are often described as groups of muscles called iliocostalis, longissimus and spinalis. The actions of the erector spinae extend (bend backwards) the spine from a flexed position to maintain a correct curvature of the spine.

Summary: in terms of sporting performance, core stability is pivotal for optimal force production and in reducing loads placed on joints in a broad spectrum of activities ranging from jumping to throwing. Analogically, a strong core is a solid foundation upon which robust structures are built; a lack of development here can see potential exposure to injury and instability. Conversely, developing this area will not only improve your overall power and speed output but also, with correct execution, protect the spine and maintain correct postural alignment, offset potential injury and amend postural imbalances, as well as enhancing functional fitness.

The core workouts in this book assist in teaching the core muscles how to engage as a unit and when to contract to stabilise and enable movement. Some of the most effective core-strengthening exercises are bodyweight exercises. *Rapid Fitness* is entirely based around these functional movements, from the squat and multi-directional lunge to the press-up – they all require the muscles of the core to stabilise and facilitate movement. Directly training these areas will improve your ability to safely and powerfully execute the workouts while simultaneously becoming mindful of engaging the core muscles when required. We need to retrain our neuromuscular system with the ability to activate our core muscles, not only on demand but also subconsciously – a function we have progressively lost through inertia and inactive lifestyles (sitting, driving, etc). Pay special attention when performing all the exercises to activate the core muscles and deliver proper stabilised movements with correct form.

CHAPTER SIX

THE EXERCISES

EXERCISE PORTFOLIO

Upper-body exercises

THE EXERCISES

Core exercises

THE EXERCISES

Pectoralis Major Clavicular Head [upper chest]

Pectoralis Major Sternal Head [lower chest]

Biceps Brachii [front of arm]

External and Internal Obliques [side of waist]

Anterior Deltoid [front of shoulder]

Lateral Deltoid [side of shoulder]

Rectus Abdominis [abs]

Erector Spinae [lower back]

Trapezius Middle and Upper Fibres [middle and upper back]

Rhomboids [middle back]

Latissimus Dorsi [middle and outer back]

Triceps Brachii [back of arms]

Quadriceps [thigh]

Adductor [inner thigh]

Transverse Abdominis [inner abs]

Soleus [small calf]

Gastrocnemius [big calf]

Gluteus Maximus [rear]

Hamstrings [rear thigh]

UPPER-BODY EXERCISES
Information on resistance training can be found on page 24.

Extended-Kneeling Press-Up
This exercise represents the easiest modification of a press-up in the book. The aim here is to build muscular strength and endurance in the chest and front of shoulders. Use this exercise as a substitute to a standard press-up if you cannot perform the prescribed repetitions. Once these become easier, you can progress onto standard press-ups.

Instructions:
A. Rest on your knees and place your hands directly below and shoulder-width apart. Maintain a straight back and engage your core.
B. Lower your torso towards the floor until your elbows form a 90° angle (keep your core engaged, avoiding sagging to the hips). Return to the start position by straightening the elbows, pushing through the palms.

Main Target: pectoralis major, sternal head (lower chest)
Secondary Target: pectoralis major, clavicular head (upper chest), anterior deltoid (front of shoulders), triceps brachii (back of arms)

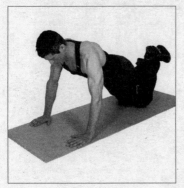 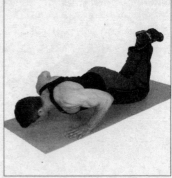

Negative Press-Up

The negative press-up focuses on the eccentric phase of the press-up (when the muscles lengthen under tension), coupled with the concentric phase (when muscles shorten under tension) of the extended-kneeling press-up. The negative press-up represents a progression from the latter and acts as a precursor to the standard press-up. Repeated use will see quick progress onto the standard press-up.

Instructions:

A. Rest on the balls of your feet, placing them hip-width apart. Position your hands directly below and shoulder-width apart. Maintain a straight line from head to heel and engage your core.

B. Lower your body very slowly towards the floor for approximately an eight-count. Keep your core engaged, avoiding sagging to the hips.

C. When almost touching the floor, drop to your knees.

D. Remain on your knees and push up your torso by straightening at the elbows.

E. Assume the original position and repeat for prescribed repetitions.

Main Target: pectoralis major, sternal head (lower chest)

Secondary Target: pectoralis major, clavicular head (upper chest), anterior deltoid (front of shoulders), triceps brachii (back of arms).

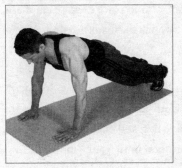 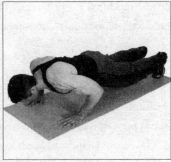

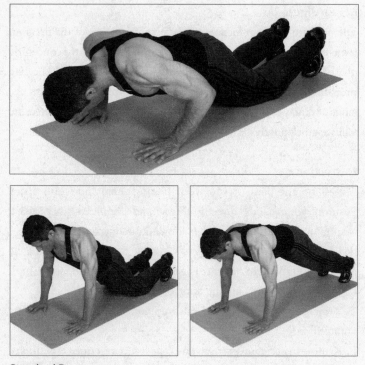

Standard Press-up

The standard press-up is the mainstay of upper-body strength conditioning. Use this exercise to build muscular strength and endurance in the chest and front of shoulders. This versatile exercise can be modified for progression and also to place exercise emphasis on different body parts, expressed through the many listed variations.

Instructions:

A. Rest on the balls of your feet, placing them hip-width apart. Position your hands directly below and shoulder-width apart. Maintain a straight line from head to heel and engage your core.

B. Lower your body towards the floor until your elbows form a

90° angle (keep your core engaged, avoiding sagging to the hips). Push back to the start position by driving through the palms and straightening the elbows.

Main Target: pectoralis major, sternal head (lower chest).
Secondary Target: pectoralis major, clavicular head (upper chest), anterior deltoid (front of shoulders), triceps brachii (back of arms).

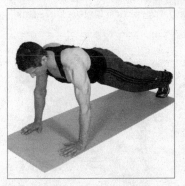
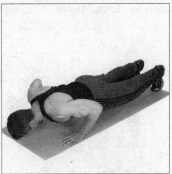

Standard Press-Up with Raised Leg

This version of the press-up presents a greater challenge than the standard version, as one leg (alternated) is held in a raised position. During the press-up, fully engage your core muscles to ensure you maintain proper form throughout the movement.

Instructions:

A. Rest on the balls of your feet, placing them hip-width apart. Position your hands directly below and shoulder-width apart. Maintain a straight line from head to heel and engage your core.

B. Lift one leg off the floor and in line with your body. To maintain the integrity of this exercise, focus on keeping the leg raised and in line while executing a perfect press-up.

C. Lower your body towards the floor until your elbows form a

90° angle (keep your core engaged, avoiding sagging to the hips). Push back to the start position by driving through the palms and straightening the elbows. Once the prescribed reps are completed, repeat with the other leg.

Main Target: pectoralis major, sternal head (lower chest)
Secondary Target: pectoralis major, clavicular head (upper chest), anterior deltoid (front of shoulders), triceps brachii (back of arms).

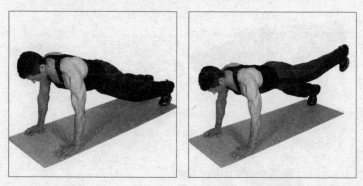

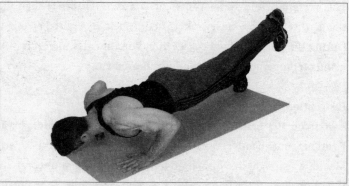

Dolphin Press-Up

The dolphin press-up is originally a yoga exercise and presents a considerable upper-body strength challenge (depending on how far you lower your body). Use the core muscles to great effect in stabilising the movement.

Instructions:
A. Begin in a plank position with the forearms shoulder-width apart, hands interlaced.
B. From this position, walk your feet forward until you reach a 90° pike position (feet remain in this advanced position).
C. Lower your body towards the floor under control (contract the core muscles to stabilise). Reverse the movement by driving back into the pike position using upper-body strength.

Main Target: pectoralis major, sternal head (lower chest), anterior deltoid (front of shoulders), triceps brachii (back of arms).
Secondary Target: pectoralis major, clavicular head (upper chest).

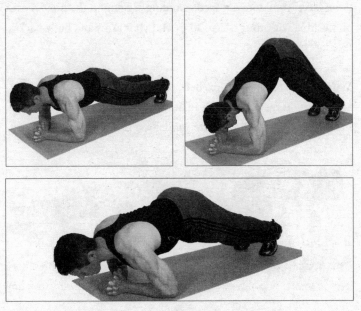

Diamond Press-Up

The diamond press-up poses a different challenge to that of the standard press-up in that more emphasis is placed on the triceps while still working the chest and front of shoulders. If this is too much of a challenge, start with the extended-kneeling press-up and modify to the diamond extended-kneeling press-up. Once mastered, you can graduate to a full diamond press-up.

Instructions:

A. Begin by kneeling on all fours and then place your thumbs and index fingers together to form a diamond, or triangle, shape.

B. Keeping your hands in this position, extend your legs, resting on the balls of your feet and hip-width apart. Maintain a straight line from head to heel and engage your core.

C. Bending at the elbows, lower your body down to just above the floor (keep your core engaged, avoiding sagging to the hips). Focus on pushing with your triceps to extend your arms and body back to the start position.

Main Target: triceps brachii (back of arms).

Secondary Target: pectoralis major, clavicular head (upper chest), sternal head (lower chest), anterior deltoid (front of shoulders).

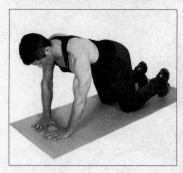 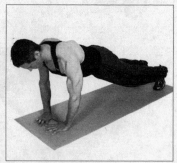

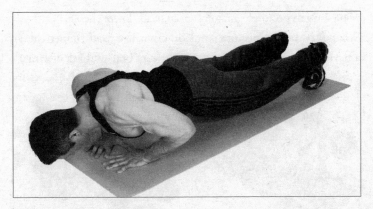

Spider-Man Press-Up

The Spider-Man press-up offers another more challenging variation on the standard press-up. This multi-joint movement activates the abdominals and hip flexors, contributing to greater core strength and co-ordination.

Instructions:

A. Rest on the balls of your feet, placing them hip-width apart. Position your hands directly below and shoulder-width apart. Maintain a straight line from head to heel and engage your core.

B. Lower your body towards the floor, simultaneously bringing your right knee towards your right elbow. When your elbows form a 90° angle (keeping your core engaged and avoiding sagging to the hips), push back to the start position by driving through the palms and straightening the elbows. Alternate legs on each rep to create a 'Spider-Man' action.

Main Target: pectoralis major, sternal head (lower chest)
Secondary Target: pectoralis major, clavicular head (upper chest), anterior deltoid (front of shoulders), triceps brachii (back of arms)

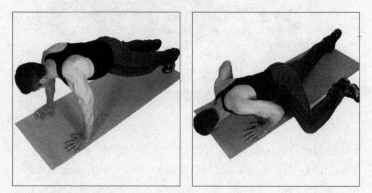

One-Handed Press-Up

The one-handed press-up is an advanced variation and involves specific attention to correct execution and full range of motion, as is mandatory with all press-ups.

Instructions:

A. Rest on the balls of your feet, placing them wider than a standard press-up, approximately twice hip-width. Position one hand directly under your body and the other behind your back. These three points of contact form a triangle. Maintain a straight line from head to heel and engage your core.

B. Lower your body towards the floor until your elbow forms a 90° angle. Pay special attention to keeping your core and glutes activated, maintaining a rigid (prone) body throughout. Push back by straightening the elbow, pushing through the palm. Alternate arms for the prescribed amount of reps.

Main Target: pectoralis major, sternal head (lower chest).
Secondary Target: pectoralis major, clavicular head (upper chest), anterior deltoid (front of shoulders), triceps brachii (back of arms).

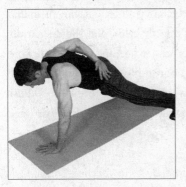 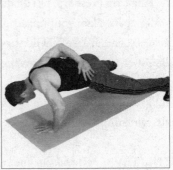

Knuckle and Fingertip Press-Ups

The knuckle press-up and fingertip press-up are very similar to the standard press-up in terms of muscles used. The focus of the knuckle press-up is to build wrist integrity, as well as strengthen the bones of the hand. In addition, the forearms are engaged more than in the standard press-up to stabilise the wrist. These are a great inclusion for combat athletes as an injury-prevention measure. The fingertip press-up focuses on the bones and muscles of the fingers and is particularly beneficial to basketball players as a preventative measure to combat jammed fingers.

Instructions:

A. **Knuckle Press-Up**: rest on the balls of your feet, placing them hip-width apart. Place your knuckles directly below and shoulder-width apart. Maintain a straight line from head to heel and engage your core.

B. Lower your body towards the floor until your elbows form a 90° angle (keep your core engaged, avoiding sagging to the hips). Push back to the start position by driving through your knuckles and straightening the elbows.

A. **Fingertip Press-Up:** rest on the balls of your feet, placing them hip-width apart. Place your fingertips directly below and shoulder-width apart. Maintain a straight line from head to heel and engage your core. B. Lower your body towards the floor until your elbows form a 90° angle (keep your core engaged, avoiding sagging to the hips). Push back to the start position by driving through your fingertips and straightening the elbows.

Main Target: pectoralis major, sternal head (lower chest).
Secondary Target: pectoralis major, clavicular head (upper chest), anterior deltoid (front of shoulders), triceps brachii (back of arms)

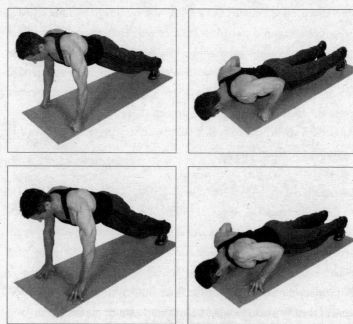

Decline Press-Up

The decline press-up is a progression up from a standard press-up, focusing on muscle strength and endurance of the upper chest.

Instructions:

A. Kneel on the floor with a chair or elevation behind you and position your hands directly below and shoulder-width apart. Place your feet on the elevation, resting on the balls. Maintain a straight line from head to heel and engage your core.

B. Lower your body towards the floor until your elbows form a 90° angle (keep your core engaged and avoid sagging to the hips). To assist complete descent, pull the head slightly back, taking care not to arch the back. Push back to the start position by driving through the palms and straightening the elbows.

Main Target: pectoralis major, clavicular head (upper chest).
Secondary Target: pectoralis major, sternal head (lower chest), anterior deltoid (front of shoulders), triceps brachii (back of arms).

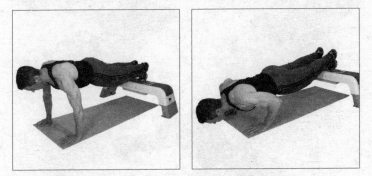

Pike Shoulder Press-Up

This focuses on muscular strength and endurance of the shoulders; one of the few exercises where direct work can be applied to them.

Instructions:

A. Start in a press-up position, placing your feet approximately twice hip-width apart and resting on the balls. Position your hands directly below and shoulder-width apart.

B. Walk your hands back, keeping your legs straight until you achieve a V-shape.

C. Lower your body towards the floor until your elbows form a 90° angle (keep your core engaged throughout). Push back to the start position by driving through the palms and straightening the elbows.

Main Target: anterior deltoid (front of shoulders).

Secondary Target: pectoralis major, clavicular head (upper chest), triceps brachii (back of arms), lateral deltoid (side of shoulders), trapezius middle and upper fibres (middle and upper back).

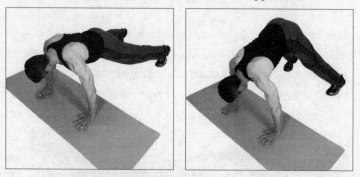

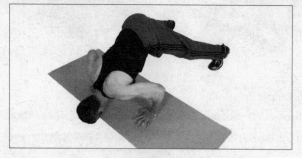

Decline Pike Shoulder Press-Up

The decline pike shoulder press-up focuses on muscular strength and endurance of the shoulders; the intensity is greater with this version as the legs are elevated.

Caution: Ensure your chosen elevation (chair, etc) is completely secure.

Instructions:

A. Start in a decline press-up position, placing your feet on a secure elevation approximately twice hip-width apart (wider if the elevation allows). Position your hands directly below and shoulder-width apart.

B. Walk your hands back, keeping your legs straight until you achieve an approximate V-shape.

C. Lower your body towards the floor until your elbows form a 90° angle (keep your core engaged throughout). Return to the start position by driving through the palms and straightening the elbows.

Main Target: anterior deltoid (front of shoulders).

Secondary Target: pectoralis major, clavicular head (upper chest), triceps brachii (back of arms), lateral deltoid (side of shoulders), trapezius middle and upper fibres (middle and upper back).

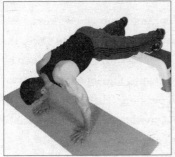 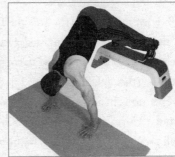

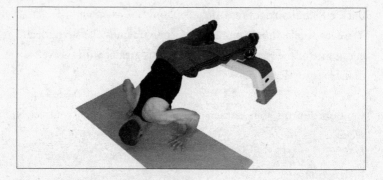

Staggered Press-Up

This presents more of a challenge than a standard press-up, as the staggered positioning of the hands creates a higher intensity and more 'load' on one arm versus the conventional press-up hand setting. This exercise is also great for balance and co-ordination, with considerable focus on stabilising.

Instructions:

A. Rest on the balls of your feet, placing them hip-width apart. Position your hands below your body in a staggered position (as they would be when walking). Make a special note to keep elbows close to the sides of the body (as opposed to flaring out to the sides as in regular press-up variations). Maintain a straight line from head to heel and engage your core.

B. Lower your body towards the floor until your elbows form a 90° angle (keep your core engaged, avoiding sagging to the hips). Keep the elbows tucked in and avoid flaring. Push back to the start position by driving through the palms and straightening the elbows. Perform two repetitions in a one-hand staggered position. Then change position and perform another two repetitions, continuing in this fashion until all prescribed repetitions have been completed.

Main Target: pectoralis major, sternal head (lower chest).
Secondary Target: pectoralis major, clavicular head (upper chest), anterior deltoid (front of shoulders), triceps brachii (back of arms)

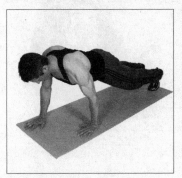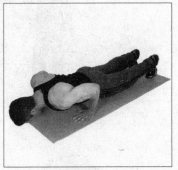

Inchworm and Press-Up

The inchworm by itself is a good warm-up exercise; coupled with a press-up, it becomes more challenging. As well as working the chest, shoulders and core muscles, there is a good stretch through the hamstrings (back of legs).

Instructions:
A. Stand with your feet hip-width apart.
B. Keep your legs straight (but bend if required) and hinge forward, flexing the spine and placing your palms flat on the floor.
C. Walk yourself forward, wrists under shoulders, keeping your core engaged.
D. When you reach press-up position, perform one repetition.
E. Reverse the process and walk the hands back to the feet, then repeat.

Main Target: pectoralis major, sternal head (lower chest).
Secondary Target: pectoralis major, clavicular head (upper chest), anterior deltoid (front of shoulders), triceps brachii (back of arms).

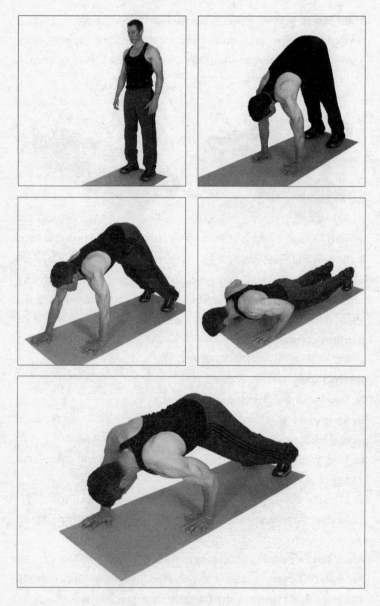

Elevated Dip

The Elevated dip targets the muscular strength and endurance of the triceps brachii (back of arms). Select an elevation that is secure, like a sturdy chair for example.

Instructions:

A. Sit on a secure elevation, placing your hands on the edge with your arms straight.

B. Slide off the elevation, keeping your legs straight and your heels on the floor.

C. Maintaining this position, lower the body by bending at the elbows to approximately 90° (or until you feel stretching on the chest or shoulders). Push back to the start position, focusing on pushing through with your triceps.

Main Target: triceps brachii (back of arms).

Secondary Target: deltoid (front of shoulders) pectoralis major, clavicular head (upper chest), sternal head (lower chest), rhomboids (middle back) and latissimus dorsi (middle/outer back).

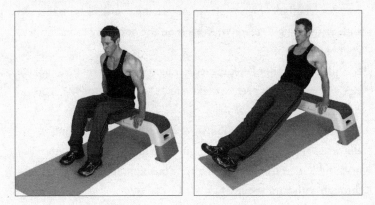

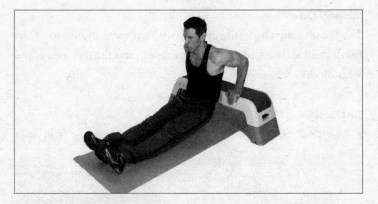

Double Elevated Dip

The double elevated dip targets the muscular strength and endurance of the triceps brachii (back of arms). This exercise represents a progression from the standard elevated dip, as both upper body and legs are raised, placing increased resistance on the triceps.

Instructions:

A. Select two forms of secure elevations (two sturdy chairs of the same height, for example). Position the second elevation just short of your leg length. Sit on one elevation, placing your hands on the edge with arms straight. Place your heels on the opposing elevation with your legs straight.

B. Slide off elevation, keeping legs straight and heels on the opposing elevation. (You may need to make a few minor adjustments to ensure correct distance and comfort).

C. Maintaining this position, lower the body by bending at the elbows to approximately 90° (or until you feel stretching on the chest or shoulders). Push back to the start position, focusing on pushing through with your triceps.

Main Target: triceps brachii (back of arms).

Secondary Target: deltoid (front of shoulders), pectoralis major, clavicular head (upper chest), sternal head (lower chest), rhomboids (middle back), latissimus dorsi (middle/outer back).

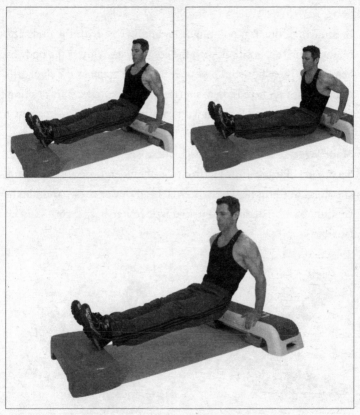

Extended Floor Dip with Leg Extension

This exercise simultaneously works both the triceps and core muscles. Special attention is given to keeping the extended leg straight throughout the range of motion, engaging your core while pushing through with the triceps.

Instructions:

A. Start by sitting on the floor. Elevate the torso by extending the arms in line with the shoulders, palms towards the floor, fingers pointing forward. The knees are bent with the lower legs perpendicular to the floor.

B. Straighten one leg, pointing it up and in line with the other leg. Maintaining this position, with the core engaged, lower the body by bending at the elbows until your rear almost touches the floor (the range of motion here is quite short). Push back to the start position, focusing on pushing through with your triceps.

Main Target: triceps brachii (back of arms).

Secondary Target: deltoid (front of shoulders), pectoralis major, clavicular head (upper chest), sternal head (lower chest), rhomboids (middle back), latissimus dorsi (middle/outer back), core muscles (various).

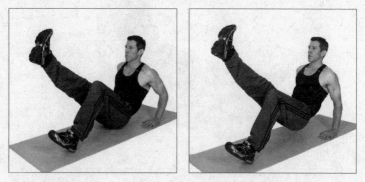

LEG EXERCISES

Information on resistance training can be found on page 24.

Standard Squat

The standard squat is a versatile compound movement (multi-joint movement) building muscular strength and endurance into the legs. Pay special attention to execute with proper form.

Note: the 'set-up' position can differ from person to person, depending on their biomechanical make-up. The most important detail is that joints are kept aligned and positioning of the feet comfortable for the individual's biomechanical movement pattern. Adjust feet until you find the ideal position before beginning the workout.

Instructions:

A. Begin with feet marginally wider apart than hip-width, knees slightly bent and toes slightly turned out. Feet, knees and hips should be aligned. The spine should be in a neutral position (natural arch) and remain this way throughout the squat. Arms can be held in front at shoulder level or across the chest.

B. Lower the body by bending forward at the knees and pushing the backside out in a sitting-down motion. Keep your knees in line with your hips and feet. Let the torso naturally tip forward from the hips, keeping your chest 'proud' as you sit back into the squat. Keep the heels down and avoid the knees coming over the toes (the exception here is when an individual has long femurs/thigh bones; in this instance knees should come over toes to maintain natural movement). Descend until your thighs are parallel (or just below). Return to the start position by pushing through the heels and extending the knees and hips until your legs are straight.

Main Target: quadriceps (thighs).
Secondary Target: gluteus maximus (rear), adductor magnus (inner thigh), soleus (small calf).

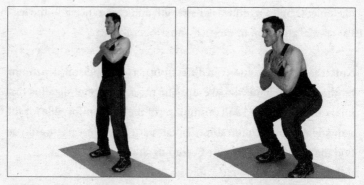

Wide Squat

The wide squat is considered a more powerful mechanical movement than the standard squat. The foot placement of one and a half times shoulder-width (or 150 per cent shoulder-width) has been observed to be the optimum spacing to generate power, with greater all-round activation of muscles fibres, including more engagement of the glutes and hips in comparison to standard squats.

Note: the 'set-up' position can differ from person to person, depending on their biomechanical make-up. The important detail is that joints are kept aligned and positioning of the feet is comfortable for the individual's biomechanical movement pattern. Adjust your feet until you find the ideal position before beginning the workout.

Instructions:

A. Begin with feet one and a half shoulder-width apart, knees slightly bent and toes slightly turned out. Feet, knees and hips should be aligned. The spine should be in a neutral position (natural arch) and remain this way throughout the squat. Arms can be held in front at shoulder level or across the chest.

B. Lower the body by bending forward at the knees and pushing the backside out in a sitting-down motion. Keep your knees in line with your hips and feet. Let the torso naturally tip forward from the hips, keeping your chest 'proud' as you sit back into the squat. Keep the heels down and avoid the knees coming over the toes. Descend until your thighs are parallel (or just below). Return to the start position by pushing through the heels and extending the knees and hips until your legs are straight.

Main Target: quadriceps (thighs).
Secondary Target: gluteus maximus (rear), adductor magnus (inner thigh), soleus (small calf).

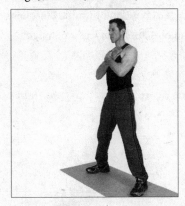 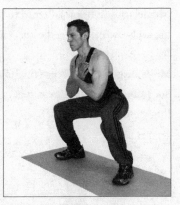

Prisoner Squat
Technically the same as the wide squat, with increased intensity due to the different hand positioning (behind the head).

Note: the 'set-up' position can differ from person to person, depending on their biomechanical make-up. The important detail is that joints are kept aligned and positioning of the feet is comfortable for the individual's biomechanical movement pattern. Adjust your feet until you find the ideal position before beginning the workout.

Instructions:

A. Begin with feet one and a half shoulder-width apart, knees slightly bent and toes slightly turned out. Keep your knees in line with your hips and feet. The spine should be in a neutral position (natural arch) and remain this way throughout the squat. Place your hands behind your head, fingers interlaced.

B. Lower the body by bending forward at the knees and pushing the backside out in a sitting-down motion. Keep your knees in line with your hips and feet. Let the torso naturally tip forward from the hips, keeping your chest 'proud' as you sit back into the squat. Keep your heels down and avoid the knees coming over the toes. Descend until your thighs are parallel (or just below). Return to the start position by pushing through the heels and extending the knees and hips until your legs are straight.

Main Target: quadriceps (thighs).

Secondary Target: gluteus maximus (rear), adductor magnus (inner thigh), soleus (small calf).

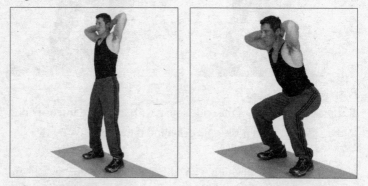

Bulgarian Squat

The Bulgarian squat is an intense squat variation. Isolating one leg at a time involves a high degree of proprioception (perception of one's own movement and spatial orientation) and co-ordination, with considerable demand placed on the core muscles and glute of the supporting leg to stabilise the movement. This single-leg strength builder is a good precursor to other, more advanced single-leg exercises like the pistol squat.

Instructions:
A. Place an elevation behind you (a stable chair, for example). Rest the ball of one foot on the elevation with hips, knees and toes in line and facing forward. The spine should be in a neutral position (natural arch) and remain this way throughout the squat. Place your hands on your hips or away from your body to counterbalance and assist stabilisation.
B. Descend by bending forward at the knee. Maintain a straight line through your body, keeping your chest 'proud'. Avoid the knee coming over the toe. Descend until your thigh is parallel (or just below parallel) with the floor and your trailing leg almost touches the floor. Return to the start position by extending the knee and hip until your leg is straight. Repeat with the opposite leg.

Main Target: quadriceps (thighs).
Secondary Target: gluteus maximus (rear), adductor magnus (inner thigh), soleus (small calf).

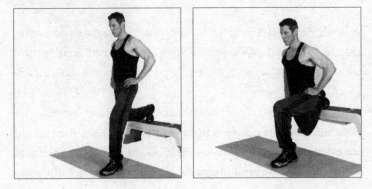

Regular and Assisted Pistol Squats

The single-leg squat, or pistol squat, represents the most intense squat in the book. If you haven't attempted a pistol squat before, you will need to build into them. First, try the Bulgarian squat and then attempt assisted pistol squats, using a stable elevation to counterbalance (a sturdy chair, for example). Partial (limited range of motion) repetitions are another easier version to build upon. There is a high degree of proprioception and co-ordination involved, with considerable demand placed on the core muscles and glute of the supporting leg to stabilise the movement.

Instructions:

A. Regular Pistol Squat: begin with your feet slightly wider apart than hip-width. The spine should begin in a neutral position (natural arch). Place your weight onto one supporting leg.

B. Descend by bending at the knee of the supporting leg (align the knee with the foot throughout the movement). Keep the opposite leg extended and as high as possible. At the bottom of the squat, the spine will flex (bend outwards) to sustain the centre of gravity. Return to the start position by extending knee and hip until your leg is straight. Repeat for prescribed repetitions and then change legs.

A. **Assisted Pistol Squat:** begin with your feet slightly wider apart than hip-width. The spine should begin in a neutral position (natural arch). Place your weight onto one supporting leg while using a stable base.

B. Descend by bending at the knee of the supporting leg (align the knee with the foot throughout the movement). Keep the opposite leg extended and as high as possible. At the bottom of the squat, the spine will flex (bend outwards) to sustain the centre of gravity.

Return to the start position by extending knee and hip until your leg is straight. Repeat for prescribed repetitions and then change legs.

Main Target: quadriceps (thighs).
Secondary Target: gluteus maximus (rear), adductor magnus (innner thigh), soleus (small calf).

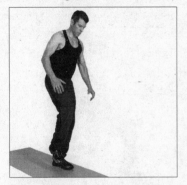 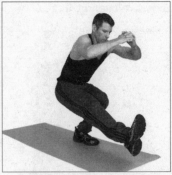

Alternate Lunge

The lunge is another compound lower-body exercise that requires excellent balance and co-ordination. The multiple planes of motion involved in this movement require considerable stabilisation, making the lunge a highly effective functional exercise (mimicking everyday and sports-specific movements). Attention to lead foot placement is important, as a longer lunge will shift the emphasis onto the gluteus.

Instructions:

A. Begin with your feet slightly wider apart than hip-width, knees slightly bent. The spine should be in a neutral position (natural arch) and remain this way throughout the lunge.

B. Take a comfortable lunge forward, landing heel to toe. Descend by bending the knee of the lead leg, keeping the torso upright throughout. Maintain alignment of the lead knee with the hip and ankle. Continue to lower the body until your trailing leg almost touches the floor. Return to the start position by powerfully extending the knee and hip. Alternate with the opposite leg for prescribed repetitions.

Main Target: quadriceps (thighs).
Secondary Target: gluteus maximus (rear), adductor magnus (inner thigh), soleus (small calf).

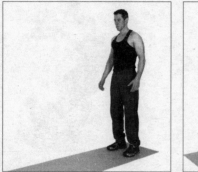 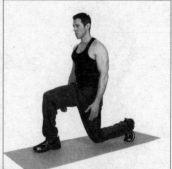

Reverse Lunge

This is exactly as described: a reverse of the standard lunge. This reversal of motion offers a different challenge in terms of co-ordination and stability. Emphasis can be placed more on the glutes by taking a longer backwards step.

Instructions:

A. Begin with your feet slightly wider apart than hip-width, knees slightly bent. The spine should be in a neutral position (natural arch) and remain this way throughout the lunge.

B. Take a comfortable step backwards, landing and remaining on the ball of your foot. Descend by bending the knee of the supporting leg, keeping the torso upright throughout. Maintain alignment of the lead knee with the hip and ankle. Continue to lower the body until your rear leg almost touches the floor. Return to the start position by extending the knee and hip of the supporting leg. Alternate with the opposite leg for prescribed repetitions.

Main Target: quadriceps (thighs).
Secondary Target: gluteus maximus (rear), adductor magnus (inner thigh), soleus (small calf).

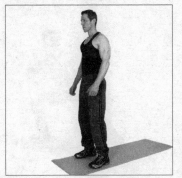 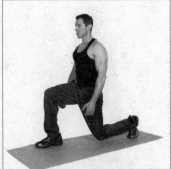

Side Lunge

The lateral movement of the side-to-side lunge places more emphasis on the adductors (muscles of the inner thigh) than the standard lunge. Benefits are to be found in co-ordination, stability and flexibility.

Instructions:
A. Begin with your feet slightly wider apart than hip-width, knees slightly bent. The spine should be in a neutral position (natural arch) and remain this way throughout the lunge.

B. Take a comfortable lunge to the side, landing heel to ball. Descend by bending the knee of the lead leg, keeping the torso upright throughout. Maintain alignment of the lead knee with the hip and ankle. Continue to lower the body until your trailing leg almost touches the floor. Return to the start position by powerfully extending the knee and hip. Alternate with the opposite leg for prescribed repetitions.

Main Target: quadriceps (thighs).
Secondary Target: gluteus maximus (rear), all adductors (magnus, longus and brevis, or inner thigh, soleus, small calf).

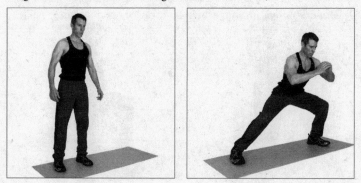

Multi-Directional Lunge

The directional lunge adds a further dimension to the standard lunge as extra emphasis is placed on the adductor muscles (inner thigh). Begin with 45°, alternating legs. Vary degrees to condition the body to multiple planes of movement. This is beneficial for sports involving multi-directional requirements and high functional benefit.

Instructions:

A. Begin with your feet slightly wider apart than hip-width, knees slightly bent. The spine should be in a neutral position (natural arch) and remain this way throughout the lunge. Place hands on hips.

B. Take a comfortable lunge forward at 45°, landing heel to ball. Descend by bending the knee of the lead leg, keeping the torso upright throughout. Maintain alignment of the lead knee with the hip and ankle. Continue to lower the body until trailing your leg almost touches the floor. Return to the start position by powerfully extending the knee and hip. Alternate with the opposite leg for prescribed repetitions.

Main Target: quadriceps (thighs).
Secondary Target: gluteus maximus (rear), all adductors (magnus, longus and brevis, or inner thigh and soleus, or small calf).

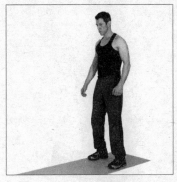 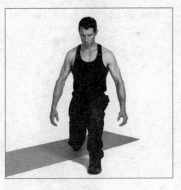

Walking Lunge

The walking lunge is a great functional exercise, working the body on multiple planes of motion, improving stabilisation and balance. The total amount of work involved in transferring weight up and down makes this version more challenging than the standard lunge.

Instructions:

A. Begin with your feet slightly wider apart than hip-width, knees slightly bent. The spine should be in a neutral position (natural arch) and remain this way throughout the lunge.

B. Take a comfortable lunge forward, landing heel to toe. Descend by bending the knee of the lead leg, keeping the torso upright throughout. Maintain alignment of the lead knee with the hip and ankle. Continue to lower the body until your trailing leg almost touches the floor.

C. Push off from the lead foot, driving the body up. Then lunge forward with the opposite leg to create a walking lunge motion. Stay upright throughout the movement. Repeat for prescribed repetitions.

Main Target: quadriceps (thighs).
Secondary Target: gluteus maximus (rear), adductor magnus (inner thigh), soleus (small calf).

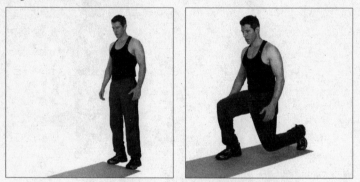

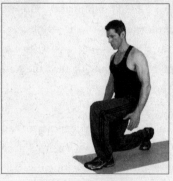

Single-Leg RDL (Romanian Deadlift)
The one-leg RDL is a challenging single-leg strength and stability exercise, popular with dancers to rebalance the muscles of the

lower legs and create extra stability when dancing. The muscular contraction focus here is on the glutes and hamstrings, with an array of stabilisers facilitating the movement.

Instructions:
A. Begin with your feet slightly wider apart than hip-width, knees slightly bent. The spine should be in a neutral position (natural arch). Assume a kick stance to put weight onto the supporting leg.

B. The aim is to bring the heel, rear and head parallel with the floor. Reach down towards the toes of the supporting leg while maintaining a neutral spine. Avoid reaching too far forward as this will round the back (flex spine). Concentrate on the contraction through the hamstring (back of leg) of the supporting leg. Return to the kick stance and repeat. Alternate with the opposite leg.

Main Target: hamstrings (rear thighs) and gluteus maximus (rear).

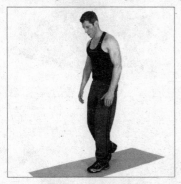 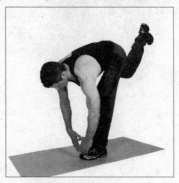

Donkey Kick to Hip Extension

The donkey kick to hip extension is a hamstring (back of leg) and hip-dominant exercise. Focus on the contraction of the hamstring and glutes, with special attention placed on the heel position throughout the range of motion.

Instructions:

A. Assume a quadrupedal position (on all fours, hands directly below the shoulders and knees hip-width apart).

B. Drop down to your elbows to avoid excessive use of the lower back. This will slightly flex the spine. However, the range of motion will bring it into neutral.

C. Donkey kick by pushing your heels up to the ceiling.

D. Extend the hips and knees, keeping your heels pointing as far back as possible (avoid pointing the toes, as the leg will drop and, instead, activate the quad).

Main Target: hamstrings (rear thigh) and gluteus maximus (rear).

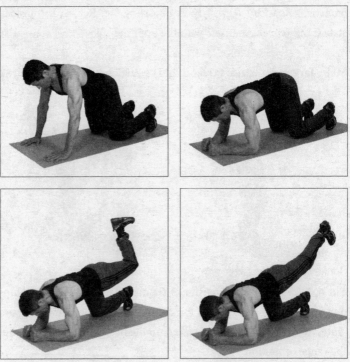

Supine Bridge and Single-Leg Bridge

The supine bridge targets glute function. This exercise is popular with runners and other types of athletes, as glute function is often a weak spot, particularly for those with existing knee or back pain. Using the supine bridge will reduce pain in these areas and work as injury prevention when going forward, removing stress from the hamstrings and lower back. Also, a huge amount of power is generated from the glutes, so more function here equals more power output. For runners and athletes, this equates to greater hip function and stride length. The concentration on glute activation teaches them to fire for improved propulsion.

Instructions:

A. Lie on your back, knees bent, feet flat and hip-width apart with arms by your side, palms facing down.

B. Push your hips up into a bridge by activating your glutes and pushing through your heels. During elevation, keep lower back muscles out of the movement (it is important not to overarch). Take care not to let the hamstrings overwork here either; focus entirely on glute activation. Perform repetitions at a slow tempo.

C. Increase the level of intensity by performing the single-leg bridge. Assume the same starting position and, this time, extend one leg.

D. As you activate the glute and drive the hips up into a bridge, keep the extended leg straight and in line with your body.

Main Target: gluteus maximus (rear).
Secondary Target: hamstrings (rear thigh).

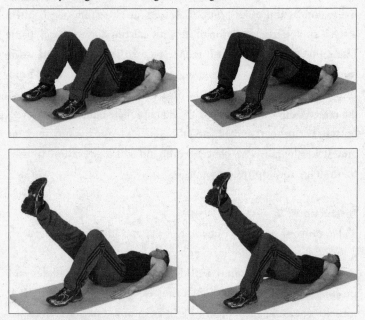

Calf Raise and Single-Leg Calf Raise

The calf raise is the only exercise in the book that targets the main component of the calf muscle: the gastrocnemius. Ideally, use an elevation (a step, for example) to facilitate a full range of motion, although these can still be performed from the floor.

Instructions:

A. Calf Raise: stand in a neutral position with your feet hip-width apart. Hands can be placed across the chest.

B. Lock the knees back, keeping your legs straight throughout the movement. Extend the ankles and raise the heels by pushing through the balls of the feet. Lower and repeat. When performed on an elevation, the feet should start in dorsiflexion (heels down with balls of feet on the edge of the step). Then extend the ankle into plantar flexion, rising up onto the balls of your feet. Repeat for prescribed repetitions.

A. Single-Leg Calf Raise: to perform the single-leg variation, set up on one foot.
B. Raise and bend one leg, following the same instructions. This will be more intense, as the single calf will bear the whole load.

Main Target: gastrocnemius (big calf).
Secondary Target: soleus (small calf).

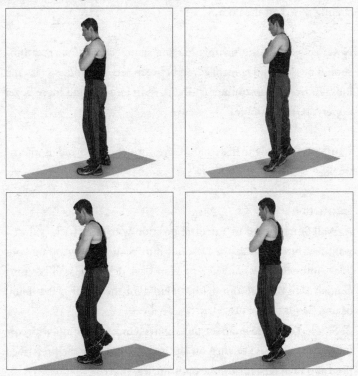

ISOMETRIC EXERCISE
Information on isometric training can be found on page 30

YIELDING ISOMETRICS

Wall Squat and Single-Leg Wall Squat
The wall squat is a powerful exercise aimed at strength-conditioning the legs and backside, popular with power-lifters and skiers. These exercises are also a good preventative measure against 'runner's knee', typically associated with weak quadriceps and tight hamstrings. To increase the level of intensity, these can be performed with one foot slightly raised off the floor.

Note: activate all motor units during static contraction. Breathing should be slow and controlled. In between sets, introduce a fast and loose movement to counteract the tension (see fast and loose boxer uppercuts, for example).

Caution: those with high blood pressure should avoid isometric work.

Instructions:
A. Wall Squat: stand in a neutral position with your back against a wall, feet hip-width apart. Descend into position by bending your knees into 90° angles and sliding your back down the wall (keeping contact with the wall throughout). Hold for the prescribed amount of time.
B. Single-Leg Wall Squat: set-up as above. Once in position, with core fully activated, raise one leg off the ground, hold for the prescribed time and then repeat with the opposite leg.

Exercise focus: increased motor-unit recruitment.

Main Target: quadriceps (thighs).

Secondary Target: gluteus maximus (rear), adductor magnus (inner thigh), soleus (small calf).

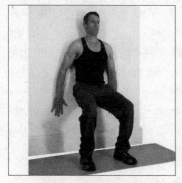 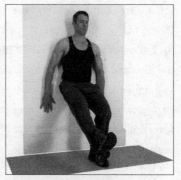

Squat Hold

The squat hold is a powerful leg and backside conditioner, involving additional core and lower-back stabilising to the wall squat. This exercise is essentially a mid-range standard-squat static hold. The angle of the squat hold (mid-range is most intense) can be varied between workouts to increase strength through ROM and to give the CNS a rest.

Note: activate all motor-units during static contraction. Breathing should be slow and controlled. In between sets, introduce a fast and loose movement to counteract the tension (see fast and loose boxer uppercuts, for example).

Caution: those with high blood pressure should avoid isometric work.

Instructions:

A. Begin with feet marginally wider apart than hip-width, knees slightly bent and toes slightly turned out. The spine should be in a neutral position (natural arch) and remain this way throughout the squat. Arms can be held in front at shoulder level or across the chest. Lower the body by bending forward at the knees and pushing the backside out in a sitting-down motion. Keep the knees in line with the hips and feet. Let the torso naturally tip forward from the hips, keeping your chest 'proud' as you sit back into the squat. Keep your heels down and avoid the knees coming over the toes. Descend until your thighs are parallel (or just below) with the floor. Maintain this position for the prescribed time.

Exercise focus: increased motor-unit recruitment.
Main Target: quadriceps (thighs).
Secondary Target: gluteus maximus (rear), adductor magnus (inner thigh), soleus (small calf).

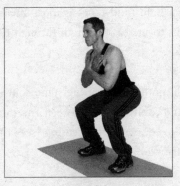

Lunge Hold

As with the squat hold, this is a mid-range static hold of the lunge. The angle of the lunge hold can be varied between workouts to increase strength through ROM and to give the CNS a rest.

THE EXERCISES

Note: activate all motor units during static contraction. Breathing should be slow and controlled. In between sets, introduce a fast and loose movement to counteract the tension (see fast and loose boxer uppercuts, for example).

Caution: those with high blood pressure should avoid isometric work.

Instructions:

Begin with your feet slightly wider apart than hip-width, knees slightly bent. The spine should be in a neutral position (natural arch) and remain this way throughout the lunge. Take a comfortable lunge forward, landing heel to toe. Descend by bending the knee of the lead leg, keeping the torso upright throughout. Maintain alignment of the lead knee with the hip and ankle. Continue to lower the body until your trailing leg almost touches the floor. Maintain this position for the prescribed time. Return to the start position and repeat with the opposite leg for the prescribed time.

Exercise focus: increased motor-unit recruitment.

Main Target: quadriceps (thighs).

Secondary Target: gluteus maximus (rear), adductor magnus (inner thigh), soleus (small calf).

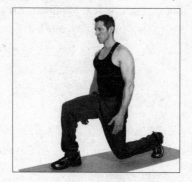

Single-Leg RDL (Romanian Deadlift) Hold

This is a mid-range static hold of the single-leg RDL. Add these for sports where lower-body strength is at a premium. The RDL hold is a highly effective exercise for stabilising and improving balance.

Note: activate all motor units during static contraction. Breathing should be slow and controlled. In between sets (one hold per leg constitutes one set), introduce a fast and loose movement to counteract the tension (see fast and loose boxer uppercuts, for example).

Caution: those with high blood pressure should avoid isometric work.

Instructions:
Begin with feet slightly wider than hip-width apart, knees slightly bent. The spine should be in a neutral position (natural arch). Assume a kick stance to put weight onto the supporting leg. The aim is to bring the heel, rear and head parallel with the floor. Reach down towards the toes of the supporting leg whilst maintaining a neutral spine. Avoid reaching too far forward, as this will round the back (flex spine). Concentrate on the contraction through the hamstring (back of leg) of the supporting leg. Maintain this position for the prescribed time. Alternate with the opposite leg.

Exercise focus: increased motor-unit recruitment.
Main Target: hamstrings (rear thigh), gluteus maximus (rear).

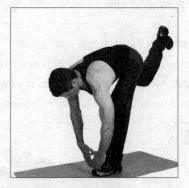

Press-Up Hold

This is a mid-range static hold of the press-up. Add these for sports where upper-body strength is at a premium. The angle of the press-up hold can be varied over workouts to increase strength through ROM and to give the CNS a rest.

Note: activate all motor units during static contraction. Breathing should be slow and controlled. In between sets, introduce a fast and loose movement to counteract the tension (see fast and loose boxer uppercuts, for example).

Caution: those with high blood pressure should avoid isometric work.

Instructions:
A. Rest on the balls of your feet, placing them hip-width apart. Position your hands directly below and shoulder-width apart. Maintain a straight line from head to heel and engage your core.

Lower your body towards the floor until your elbows form a 90° angle (keep your core engaged, avoiding sagging to the hips). Maintain this position for the prescribed time.

Exercise focus: increased motor-unit recruitment.
Main Target: pectoralis major, sternal head (lower chest).
Secondary Target: pectoralis major, clavicular head (upper chest), anterior deltoid (front of shoulders), triceps brachii (back of arms).

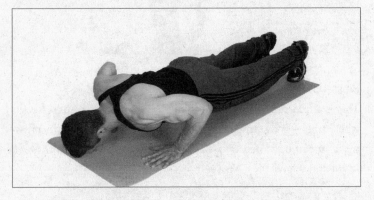

Pike Shoulder-Press Hold

This is a mid-range static hold of the pike shoulder press. Add these for sports where upper-body strength is at a premium. The angle can be varied over workouts to increase strength through ROM and to give the CNS a rest.

Note: activate all motor units during static contraction. Breathing should be slow and controlled. In between sets, introduce a fast and loose movement to counteract the tension (see fast and loose boxer uppercuts, for example).

Caution: those with high blood pressure should avoid isometric work.

Instructions:

Start in a pike shoulder-press position, placing your feet approximately twice hip-width apart and resting on the balls. Position your hands directly below and shoulder-width apart. Walk your hands back, keeping your legs straight until you achieve a V-shape. Lower your body towards the floor until your elbows form a 90° angle (keep the core engaged throughout). Maintain this position for the prescribed time.

Exercise focus: increased motor-unit recruitment.

Main Target: anterior deltoid (front of shoulders).

Secondary Target: pectoralis major, clavicular head (upper chest), triceps brachii (back of arms), lateral deltoid (side of shoulder), trapezius middle and upper fibres (middle and upper back).

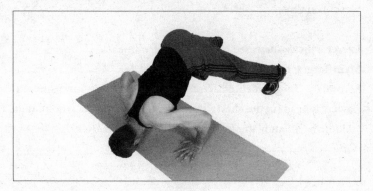

Elevated Dip Hold

This is a mid-range static hold of the elevated dip. Add these for sports where upper-body strength is at a premium. The angle can be varied over workouts to increase strength through ROM and to give the CNS a rest.

Note: activate all motor units during static contraction. Breathing should be slow and controlled. In between sets, introduce a fast and loose movement to counteract the tension (see fast and loose boxer uppercuts, for example).

Caution: those with high blood pressure should avoid isometric work.

Instructions:
Sit on a secure elevation, placing your hands on the edge with your arms straight. Slide off the elevation, keeping your legs straight and your heels on the floor. Maintaining this position, lower the body by bending at the elbows to approximately 90° (or until you feel stretching on the chest or shoulders). Maintain this position for the prescribed time.

Exercise focus: increased motor-unit recruitment.
Main Target: triceps brachii (back of arms).
Secondary Target: deltoid (front of shoulders), pectoralis major, clavicular head (upper chest), sternal head (lower chest), rhomboids (middle back) and latissimus dorsi (middle/outer back).

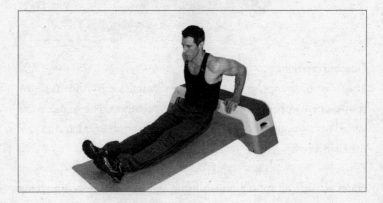

OVERCOMING ISOMETRICS

Wall Chest Press

This requires a maximal short contraction of between six and ten seconds. The resultant adaptations in strength over time are considerable and lead to abiding pectoral strength gains. Although it's impossible to measure gains during the exercise itself, you will feel the benefits when performing other chest-centric activities.

Note: maximal static contraction of six-to-ten seconds. Breathing should be slow and controlled. In between sets, introduce a fast and loose movement to counteract the tension (see fast and loose boxer uppercuts, for example).

Caution: those with high blood pressure should avoid isometric work.

Instructions:

Stand in a neutral stance approximately two feet from a wall. Drop forward, placing your palms flat on the wall with your elbows forming a 90° angle (mid-range press-up position). Adjust your stance into a staggered position, bend your left leg and bring it closer to the wall. Extend your right leg behind to create a stable platform from which to push. Take a few seconds to lead into maximal contraction and then push through your palms as hard as possible for the prescribed time. Although you are contracting every motor unit to its capacity, the focal point of intensity is through the chest.

Exercise focus: increased motor-unit recruitment.

Main Target: pectoralis major, sternal head (lower chest).

Secondary Target: pectoralis major, clavicular head (upper chest), anterior deltoid (front of shoulders) and triceps brachii (back of arms)

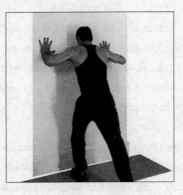

Wall Shoulder Press

This requires a maximal short contraction of between six and eight seconds. The resultant adaptations in strength over time are considerable and lead to abiding shoulder-strength gains. Although it's impossible to measure gains during the exercise itself, you will feel the benefits when performing other shoulder-centric activities.

Note: maximal static contraction of six-to-ten seconds. Breathing should be slow and controlled. In between sets, introduce a fast and loose movement to counteract the tension (see fast and loose boxer uppercuts, for example).

Caution: those with high blood pressure should avoid isometric work.

Instructions:

Stand in a neutral stance approximately three feet from a wall. Drop forward, placing your palms flat on the wall. Arms should be extended with a slight bend (20°). Adjust your stance into a staggered position, bend your left leg and bring it closer to the wall. Extend your right leg behind to create a stable platform from which to push. Drop your head in line with your spine. Take a few seconds to lead into maximal contraction and then push through your palms as hard as possible for the prescribed time. Although you are contracting every motor unit to its capacity, the focal point of intensity is through the shoulders.

Exercise focus: increased motor-unit recruitment.
Main Target: anterior deltoid (front of shoulders).
Secondary Target: pectoralis major, clavicular head (upper chest), triceps brachii (back of arms), lateral deltoid (side of shoulder), trapezius, middle and upper fibres (middle and upper back).

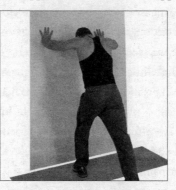

Staged Boxer Press

The aim of the staged boxer press is to improve strength at the angle of the joint through the entire ROM of a punch. In theory, this concept could be adapted to other sport-specific movements with a bit of ingenuity. Below are two staged-punch variations: the left jab and the right cross. It is advisable to use a glove (preferably a boxing glove) as the pressure exerted may create discomfort.

Note: maximal static contraction of six-to-ten seconds. Breathing should be slow and controlled. In between sets, introduce a fast and loose movement to counteract the tension (see fast and loose boxer uppercuts, for example).

Caution: those with high blood pressure should avoid isometric work.

Instructions (Left Jab):

A. Facing a wall, assume an orthodox boxer's stance (reverse these instructions if you are left-handed). From a neutral stance, take a comfortable step forward with your left leg. Angle your feet at 45° and distribute your weight with 50 per cent on each leg. Raise your hands into a cage position, elbows and chin tucked, shoulders level. Assume the initial phase of the jab (as in image), hand pressed against a wall. Once in position, rapidly build into maximal contraction.

B. Next, recreate the second phase of the jab (as in image). Assume position by edging a little further away from the wall and bending at the elbow. Once in position, rapidly build into maximal contraction.

C. To create the final phase of the jab (as in image), adjust your position further away from the wall, extend the left arm and maintain a slight angle at the elbow (approximately 20°). Your wrist should be flat with your palm facing down. Assume this position with the knuckles flat against the wall (if you have a glove of any sort, use it). Once in position, rapidly build into maximal contraction then push through the hand and arm.

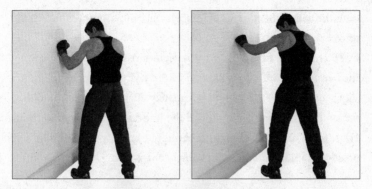

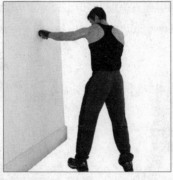

Instructions (Right Cross):

A. Facing a wall, assume an orthodox boxer's stance (reverse these instructions if you are left-handed); from a neutral stance, take a comfortable step forward with your left leg. Angle your feet at 45° and distribute your weight with 50 per cent on each leg. Raise your hands into a cage position, elbows and chin tucked, shoulders level. Assume the initial phase of the right cross (as in image), hand pressed against a wall. Once in position, rapidly build into maximal contraction.

B. Next, create the second phase of the right cross (as in image). Assume position by edging a little further away from the wall and bending at the elbow. Begin to swivel the hips, twist the torso and rise onto the ball of the foot (as in image). Once in position, rapidly build into maximal contraction.

C. To create the final phase of the right cross, adjust your position further away from the wall, extend the right arm and maintain a slight angle at the elbow (approximately 20°). Your wrist should be flat with your palm facing down, the knuckles flat against the wall. Hips, torso and ball of right foot should be fully rotated. Once in position, rapidly build into maximal contraction.

Exercise Focus: educating the body to recruit maximal motor units; building strength through the stages of a movement.

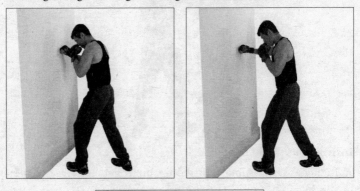

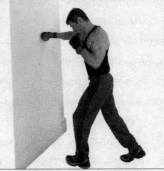

PLYOMETRIC EXERCISES

UPPER BODY

Extended-Kneeling Plyometric Press-Up

Low Intensity: this exercise represents the easier version of a plyometric press-up. The aim here is to develop upper-body power. It is a great exercise not only for combat athletes but also for throwing sports (javelin, discus, etc). Once you are accustomed to this discipline, progress onto the full plyometric press-up.

Note: focus on speed; push as fast and hard as possible away from the ground.

Caution: ensure handclap is rapid and hands are returned to start position to avoid collision with the ground.

Instructions:
A. Rest on your knees and place your hands directly below, shoulder-width apart. Maintain a straight back and engage the core and cross your feet.
B. Lower the torso towards the floor until the elbows form a 90° angle (keep the core engaged, avoiding sagging to the hips).
C. Explosively push body up and away from the floor. Rapidly clap the hands and return to the start position. Immediately drop into another press-up and repeat the process for prescribed repetitions and sets.

Exercise Target: develop upper-body power.

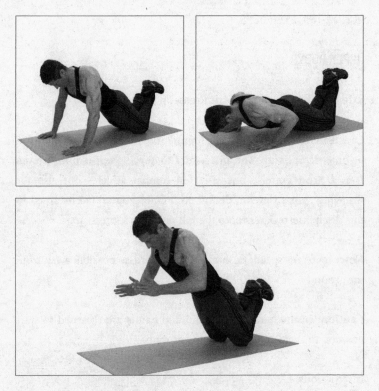

Handclap Plyometric Press-Up

Medium Intensity: the aim here is to develop upper-body power. It is a great exercise not only for combat athletes but also for throwing sports (javelin, discus, etc).

Note: focus on speed; push as fast and hard as possible away from the ground.
Caution: ensure handclap is rapid and hands are quickly returned to the start position to avoid collision with the ground.

Instructions:

A. Rest on the balls of your feet, placing them hip-width apart. Position your hands directly below and shoulder-width apart. Maintain a straight line from head to heel and engage your core.

B. Lower the torso towards the floor until the elbows form a 90° angle (keep the core engaged, avoiding sagging to the hips).

C. Explosively push the body up and away from the floor. Rapidly clap the hands and return to the start position. Immediately drop into another press-up and repeat the process for prescribed repetitions and sets.

Exercise Target: develop upper-body power.

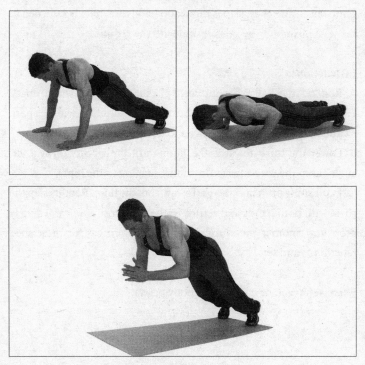

Chest-Slap Plyometric Press-Up

Medium Intensity: the chest-slap plyometric press-up is more challenging than the handclap version, as the hands have to travel a greater distance to the chest and back, requiring super rapidity in execution. The aim here is to develop upper-body power. It is a great exercise not only for combat athletes but also for throwing sports (javelin, discus, etc).

Note: focus on speed; push as fast and hard as possible away from the ground.

Caution: ensure chest slap is rapid and hands are quickly returned to the start position to avoid collision with the ground.

Instructions:
A. Rest on the balls of your feet, placing them hip-width apart. Position your hands directly below and shoulder-width apart. Maintain a straight line from head to heel and engage your core.
B. Lower the torso towards the floor until the elbows form a 90° angle (keep the core engaged, avoiding sagging to the hips).
C. Explosively push body up and away from the floor. Rapidly slap the chest with both hands and return to the start position. Immediately drop into another press-up and repeat the process for prescribed repetitions and sets.

Exercise Target: develop upper-body power.

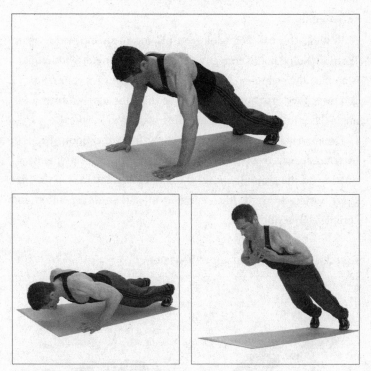

Full-Body Plyometric Press-Up

High Intensity: the aim here is to develop upper-body power. It is a great exercise not only for combat athletes but also for throwing sports (javelin, discus, etc).

Note: focus on speed; push as fast and hard as possible away from the ground, with additional emphasis placed on core muscles to assist in elevation.

Caution: this is an advanced plyometric. Become accustomed to early-stage plyometric press-ups before attempting these.

Instructions:

A. Rest on the balls of your feet, placing them hip-width apart. Position your hands directly below and shoulder-width apart. Maintain a straight line from head to heel and engage your core.

B. Lower the torso towards the floor until the elbows form a 90° angle (keep the core engaged, avoiding sagging to the hips).

C. Explosively push body up and away from the floor, using an extremely engaged core to assist entire body elevation – momentarily floating off the ground. Engage the core on landing to stop the hips from coming forward. Move straight into the next repetition and complete prescribed quota.

Exercise Target: develop upper-body power.

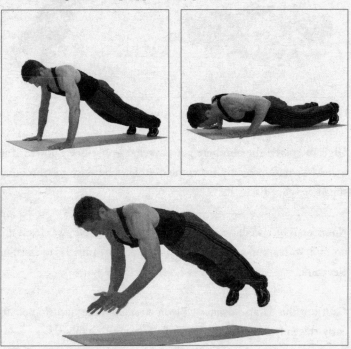

Full-Body Plyometric Press-Up to Squat

Ultra-High Intensity: this exercise combines both upper- and lower-body explosiveness in one – an extremely advanced movement. The transition from plyometric press-up into squat requires considerable power and co-ordination.

Note: focus on speed; push as fast and hard as possible away from the ground, immediately snapping hips forward and feet under.

Caution: this is an advanced plyometric. Become accustomed to early-stage plyometric press-ups before attempting.

Instructions:

A. Rest on the balls of your feet, placing them hip-width apart. Position your hands directly below and shoulder-width apart. Maintain a straight line from head to heel and engage your core.

B. Lower the torso towards the floor until the elbows form a 90° angle (keep the core engaged, avoiding sagging to the hips).

C. Explosively push body up and away from the floor, using an extremely engaged core to assist entire body elevation.

D. As the body rises, rapidly activate the hip flexors and tuck the knees to the chest, simultaneously bringing the feet to land under the body.

E. The landing position is a deep squat. Hold the position momentarily and then repeat for repetitions and sets.

Exercise Target: develop upper-body and lower-body power.

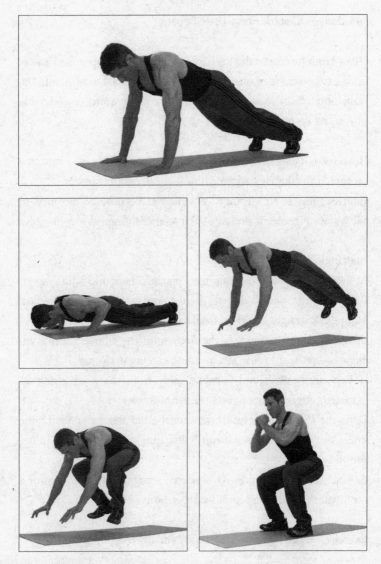

Boxing Drill – Fast and Loose Uppercuts

Low Intensity: this drill is all about co-ordination and speed. Depending on the intensity, the exercises are good for warm-ups, keeping loose between isometric drills or at a higher intensity for Tabata or GPP workouts.

Note: maintain a fluid and rhythmical movement.

Instructions:
A. Stand square on (not in boxing stance), feet shoulder-width apart, with arms in a cage position.
B. Come up onto the balls of your feet and quickly transfer your weight from one foot to the other (left-right-left-right).
C. When introducing the uppercuts, create a rolling motion with palms facing inwards. The left hand should be thrown in time with the left foot landing, the right hand with the right foot landing. Put together, this will create a smooth, co-ordinated action.

Exercise Target: develop co-ordination and explosive speed.

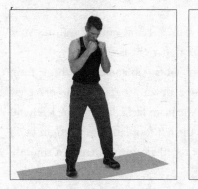 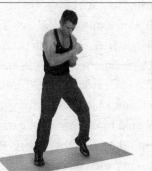

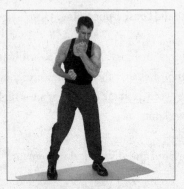

Boxing Drill – Fast and Loose Straight Shots

Low Intensity: this drill is all about co-ordination and speed. Depending on the intensity, the exercises are good for warm-ups, keeping loose between isometric drills or at a higher intensity for Tabata or GPP workouts.

Note: maintain a fluid and rhythmical movement.

Instructions:

A. Stand square on (not in boxing stance), feet shoulder-width apart, with arms in a cage position.

B. Come up onto the balls of your feet and quickly transfer your weight from one foot to the other (left-right-left-right).

C. When introducing the straight shots (jab and cross), throw from the chin, straight ahead (imagine down a barrel) in a corkscrew motion, so the wrist is flat with the palm facing down. The left hand should be thrown in time with the left foot landing, the right hand with the right foot landing. Put together, this will create a smooth, co-ordinated action.

Exercise Target: develop co-ordination and explosive speed.

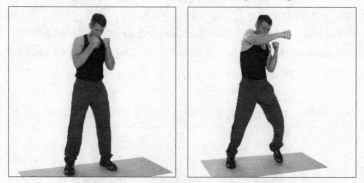

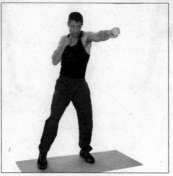

LOWER BODY

Boxing Shuffle

Low Intensity: the boxing shuffle conditions the lower body to shift weight rapidly from foot to foot, developing reaction time, co-ordination and timing.

Instructions:
A. Set-up in a boxer's stance (orthodox: left foot, left hand forward; southpaw: right foot, right hand forward) with hands in a cage

position. Distribute weight evenly on both legs. Come up onto the balls of your feet.

B. Rapidly alternate foot position, shifting back and forth continuously. Keep elbows tucked in and hands in a cage. Continue for the prescribed time.

Exercise Target: reactive strength; develop horizontal (plane) power.

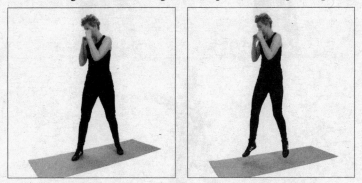

Jumping Jack

Low Intensity: the Jumping Jack is a low-intensity plyometric, suitable for multiple repetitions or set time periods. This type of plyometric offers a good platform when accustoming the body to the potential rigours of more advanced dynamic-resistance exercises. The Jumping Jack is generally considered to be a callisthenic (a general term for bodyweight) exercise. However, it's included within the plyometric list due to its explosive nature and power-development qualities.

Instructions:

A. Start in a neutral stance with feet together and arms by the sides.

B. Hop the feet out laterally while simultaneously raising your arms above your head, keeping a slight bend in the arms.

C. Quickly hop the feet back together, lowering the arms back to the sides. Repeat this motion for prescribed repetitions or time period.

Exercise Target: reactive strength; develop vertical power; conditioning precursor for more advanced exercises.

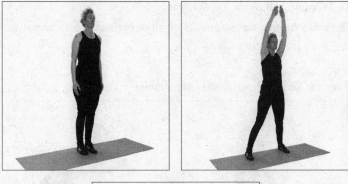

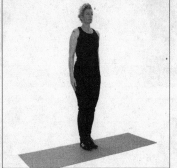

Tuck Jump

Medium Intensity: the tuck jump is suitable for single or multiple continuous repetitions or set time periods (the intensity is higher when continuous). This type of plyometric offers a good platform when accustoming the body to the potential rigours of more advanced dynamic-resistance exercises.

Instructions:

A. Start in a neutral stance with feet hip-width apart.

B. Bend at the knees and hips and drop into a half-squat.

C. From this position, explode vertically using the arms to drive momentum.

D. Ascending, draw the knees towards the chest.

E. Land on both feet and drop into the half-squat and repeat the sequence for prescribed repetitions.

Exercise Target: Reactive strength; develop vertical jump power.

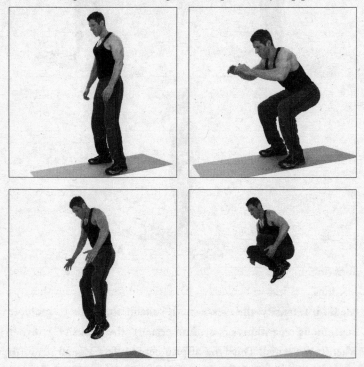

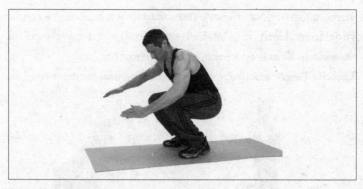

Squat Jump

Medium Intensity: the squat jump is suitable for single or multiple repetitions or set time periods (the intensity is higher when continuous). This type of plyometric offers a good platform when accustoming the body to the potential rigours of more advanced dynamic-resistance exercises.

Instructions:

A. Begin with feet marginally wider apart than hip-width, knees slightly bent and toes slightly turned out. The spine should be in a neutral position (straight back/natural arch) and remain this way throughout the squat. Hold the hands beside the head.

B. Lower the body by bending forward at the knees and pushing the backside out in a sitting-down motion. Keep the knees in line with the hips and feet. Let the torso naturally tip forward from the hips, keeping your chest 'proud' as you sit back into the squat. Keep your heels down and avoid the knees coming over the toes. Descend until your thighs are parallel with the floor.

C. From this position, explode vertically, landing back on your heels. Drop immediately into another squat and repeat for prescribed repetitions. Keep the core engaged throughout.

Exercise Target: reactive strength; develop vertical jump power.

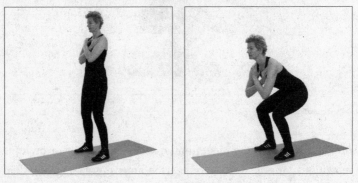

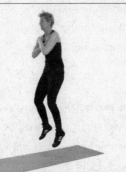

Side-to-Side Wide Squat

Low Intensity: this provides the benefits of the wide squat while introducing lateral-movement conditioning stabilisers. This exercise is suitable for multiple repetitions or set time periods. This type of plyometric offers a good platform when accustoming the body to the potential rigours of more advanced dynamic-resistance exercises.

Instructions:

A. Begin with feet one and a half shoulder-width apart, knees slightly bent and toes slightly turned out. The spine should be in a neutral position (natural arch) and remain this way throughout the squat. Arms can be held in front at shoulder level or across the chest.

B. Lower the body by bending forward at the knees and pushing the backside out in a sitting-down motion. Keep the knees in line with the hips and feet. Let the torso naturally tip forward from the hips, keeping your chest 'proud' as you sit back into the squat. Keep your heels down and avoid the knees coming over the toes. Descend until thighs are parallel (or just below). Push back to the start position.

C. From here, skip to the right, letting the left foot knock onto the right and back down into another squat.

D. Complete another squat and then skip to the left. Continue the sequence for prescribed repetitions or time period.

Exercise Target: reactive strength; develop horizontal and lateral (plane) power.

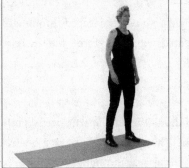 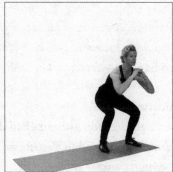

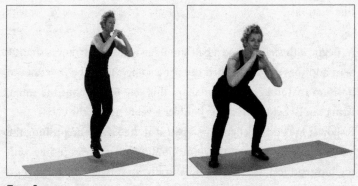

Frog Jump

Medium Intensity: the frog jump incorporates the mechanically powerful movement of the wide squat, coupled with unorthodox arm positioning. The net result creates increased focus on the hamstrings, glutes and calves to facilitate movement. Perform in single or multiple continuous repetitions (the intensity is higher when continuous).

Note: maintain focus on exploding into the jump, then landing softly into the deep squat.

Caution: concentrate on keeping core muscles engaged throughout and your back straight. If executed with poor form, this exercise could lead to discomfort or injury.

Instructions:
A. Begin with feet one and a half shoulder-width apart, knees slightly bent and toes slightly turned out. The spine should be in a neutral position (natural arch) and remain this way throughout the jump.
B. Lower the body by bending forward at the knees and pushing the backside out in a sitting-down motion. Keep your knees in line with

the hips and feet. Let the torso naturally tip forward from the hips, keeping your chest 'proud' as you sit back into a deep squat. Keep your heels down and avoid the knees coming over the toes. Descend until you assume the 'frog' position, with your hands almost touching the floor.

C. From the frog position, explode vertically.

D. Land softly and straight back into a deep squat (frog position with hands) and repeat for prescribed repetitions.

Exercise Target: reactive strength; develop vertical power.

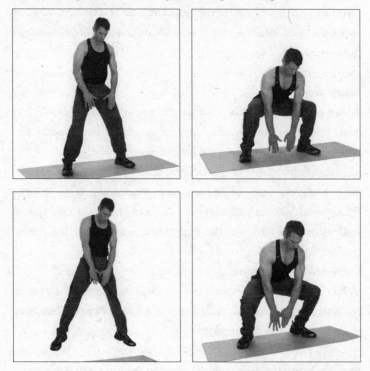

Lunge Jump

Medium Intensity: the lunge jump, as with the lunge, develops excellent balance, co-ordination and flexibility in the hips (hip flexors). The lunge jump borrows the level functionality of the lunge, coupled with the increased power of a vertical jump and leg transition, challenging dynamic stability as well as proprioception.

Note: focus on stabilising, co-ordination and quick transitions.

Caution: prior to attempting the lunge jump, first become accustomed to the standard lunge, paying special attention to co-ordination and proprioception.

Instructions:
A. Begin with feet slightly wider than hip-width apart, knees slightly bent. The spine should be in a neutral position (natural arch) and remain this way throughout the lunge.
B. Take a comfortable lunge forward, landing heel to toe. Descend by bending the knee of the lead leg, keeping the torso upright throughout. Maintain alignment of the lead knee with the hip and ankle. Continue to lower the body until your trailing leg almost touches the floor.
C. Powerfully jump vertically, extending the knees and hips.
D. Rapidly switch the position of the legs and land in a reverse position. Keep the torso upright and core engaged. Repeat alternating jumps for prescribed repetitions.

Exercise Target: reactive strength; develop vertical jump power.

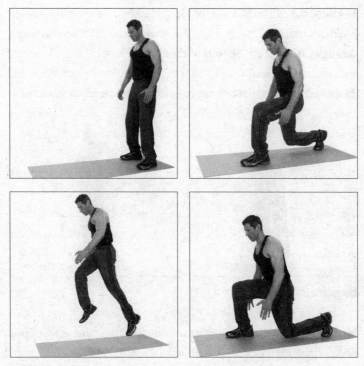

Ankle Jump

Medium Intensity: the ankle jump places emphasis on the reactive strength of the calf muscles, bolstering ability in the vertical jump and, in turn, benefiting speed and sprinting ability. These are performed continuously.

Note: maintain slight flexion of the knee and focus on generating power through the calves.

Instructions:
A. Start by standing in a neutral position. Hands on hips.

B. Using the calf muscles, explode vertically, extending the ankles. Maintain minimal flexion of the knee. Keep the core engaged throughout. Land on the balls of the feet and repeat.

Exercise Target: reactive strength; develop vertical jump powernd

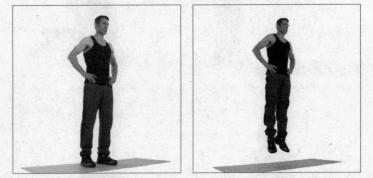

Burpee

Medium Intensity: the burpee is one of the most challenging bodyweight exercises in that it involves both upper- and lower-body anaerobic endurance. This multi-joint, explosive and highly functional exercise is popular with athletes of all levels, virtually all team sports and even with elite military forces. Its portable nature and complete design make this an ultimate conditioning exercise. Burpees are an essential component of any high-intensity program creation. The burpee is generally considered to be a callisthenic (a general term for bodyweight) exercise. However, it's included within the plyometric list due to its explosive nature and power-development qualities.

Note: focus on speed; push as fast and hard as possible away from the ground.

THE EXERCISES

Instructions:

A. Assume a press-up position.

B. Draw both feet rapidly into a squat position.

C. Explode vertically from the squat position, reaching as high as possible.

D. Land on ball to heel and drop into the squat position, kick legs back into the press-up position and repeat the process for repetitions or prescribed time period.

Exercise Target: reactive strength; develop vertical jump power.

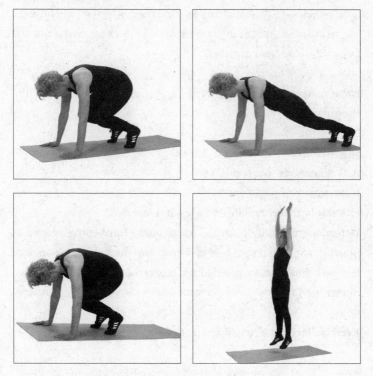

121

Burpee with Press-Up

Medium-High Intensity: the burpee with press-up is a more challenging exercise than the basic burpee, engaging the upper body to a greater extent. This multi-joint, explosive and highly functional exercise is popular with athletes of all levels, virtually all team sports and even with elite military forces. Its portable nature and complete design make this an ultimate conditioning exercise. They are an essential component of any high-intensity program creation. The burpee with press-up is generally considered to be a callisthenic (a general term for bodyweight) exercise. However, it's included within the plyometric list due its explosive nature and power-development qualities.

Note: focus on speed; push as fast and hard as possible away from the ground.

Instructions:
A. Assume a press-up position.
B. Perform one press-up.
C. Draw both feet rapidly into a squat position.
D. Explode vertically from the squat position, reaching as high as possible. Land on ball to heel and drop into the squat position, kick legs back into press-up position and repeat the process for repetitions or time period.

Exercise Target: reactive strength; develop vertical jump power.

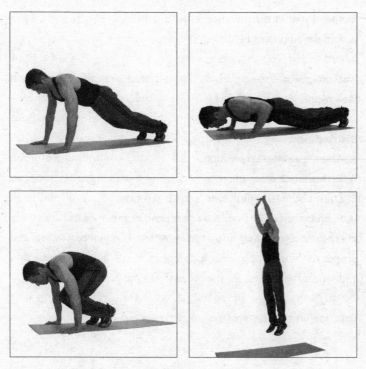

Burpee with Press-Up and Tuck Jump

High Intensity: the burpee with press-up and tuck jump is a complex, challenging bodyweight exercise in that it involves both upper- and lower-body anaerobic endurance. This multi-joint, explosive and highly functional exercise is popular with athletes of all levels, virtually all team sports and even with elite military forces. Its adaptable nature and self-contained design make this the ultimate conditioning exercise. The exercises are an essential component of any high-intensity program creation. The burpee with press-up and tuck jump is generally considered to be a callisthenic (a general term for bodyweight) exercise. However, it's included within the plyometric list due to its explosive nature and power-development qualities.

Note: focus on speed; push as fast and hard as possible away from the ground.

Instructions:
A. Assume a press-up position.
B. Perform one press-up.
C. Draw both feet rapidly into a squat position.
D. Explode vertically from the squat position; then quickly draw the knees towards the chest into a tuck position. Land on ball to heel and drop into the squat position, kick legs back into a press-up position and repeat the process for the prescribed time period.

Exercise Target: reactive strength; develop vertical jump power.

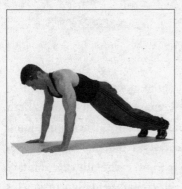 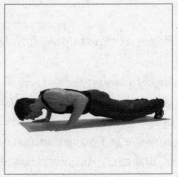

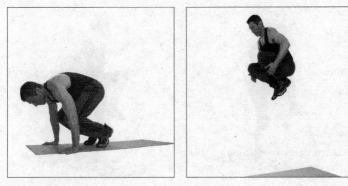

High Knees

Low-Medium Intensity: there are many different interpretations of the high-knee exercise. This version will focus on the sprinting action, using a big arm swing and high front-knee flexion with full glute extension to mimic a sprint-specific movement pattern.

Note: focus on bringing the front knee as high as possible (hence high-knee flexion and glute extension). Use a big arm swing.

Instructions:
A. Set up from a loaded running position: weight on the left foot, right knee up, left arm cocked forward and right arm behind.
B. Quickly reverse the action by bringing the right knee down and left knee up, driving the right arm forward and left arm backwards. Ensure that each knee is brought as high as possible, which in turn fully extends the glute. Stay on the balls of your feet throughout, quickly reversing the action from one side to the other.

Exercise Target: reactive strength; develop horizontal (plane) power.

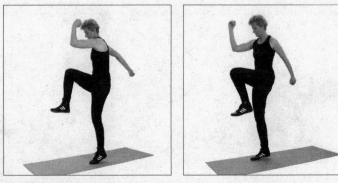

Mountain Climber

Medium Intensity: the Mountain Climber is generally considered to be a callisthenic (a general term for bodyweight) exercise but it's included within the plyometrics list due to its explosive nature. This exercise is a powerful, multi-muscle group worker. Considerable contribution is made by the core to fix the torso in place during the movement, facilitating rapid feet exchange. The Mountain Climber can be used as a warm-up exercise or as a main component to a workout, as the intensity can be easily managed.

Instructions:
A. Set up from a loaded crouching position on the balls of your feet, hands slightly wider apart than shoulder-width, with one leg flexed under the body and the other leg extended behind. Engage the core muscles.
B. Quickly exchange leg positions by extending the flexed leg and flexing the extended leg. The hips will be pushed up as the feet land simultaneously.

Exercise Target: reactive strength; develop horizontal (plane) power.

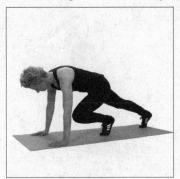 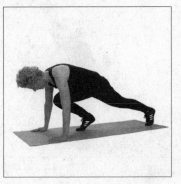

Standing Vertical Hop

Medium-High Intensity: the standing vertical hop is particularly beneficial to basketball and football (soccer) players, not only for developing lower-body explosive power but also in training the stabilisers of the hip and ankle, helping to protect the knees.

Note: concentrate on exploding as fast and as high as possible into the jump.

Instructions:
A. Set up from a loaded position, standing on your left leg.
B. Push off with the left foot with maximum power, using the right knee and arm swing to propel upwards.
C. Land ball to heel. Continue for prescribed repetitions and sets.

Exercise Target: reactive strength; develop vertical-jump power.

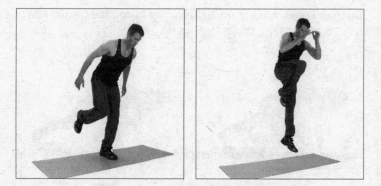

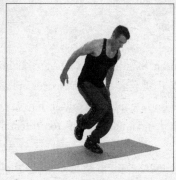

Standing Long Jump

Medium Intensity: this exercise improves horizontal jumping ability and contributes to sprinting power, as the training focus is on the horizontal plane. Pay attention to co-ordinating arm swings with the lower body to produce forward drive. These are to be performed in single repetitions.

Note: focus on exploding in the quickest possible time, jumping fast and as far as possible. Concentrate on stabilising with the hips and ankles on landing.

Instructions:

A. Assume a standing long-jump position. Keep your chest over your knees and your knees over your feet.

B. Create momentum with the arms.

C. Explode forwards into the long jump. Land on the soles of your feet (flatfooted) softly and into a squat position.

Exercise Target: reactive strength; develop horizontal (plane) power.

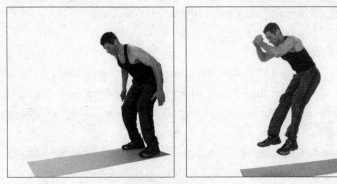

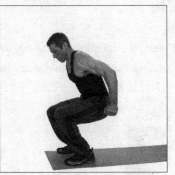

Forward Single-Leg Hop

Medium-High Intensity: the forward single-leg hop is particularly beneficial to basketball players, not only for developing lower-body explosive power but also in training the stabilisers of the hip and ankle, helping to protect the knees. This exercise will focus on a hop-stabilise sequence as opposed to continual hopping (which can be adopted if preferred).

Note: focus on exploding into the hop, then landing and stabilising without taking an extra step. To convert the hop-stabilise sequence into a continuous hop sequence, land on the ball of the foot, making minimal contact before exploding into the next hop.

Instructions:
A. Set up from a loaded position, standing on your left leg
B. Push off with the left foot with maximum power, using the right leg and arm swing to propel forwards and upwards. Keep your body straight.
C. Land on the sole (flatfooted) of the left foot and stabilise without taking any extra steps. Continue for prescribed hops and then repeat with the opposite leg.

Exercise Target: reactive strength: develop horizontal jump power; develop ability to decelerate and stabilise under control.

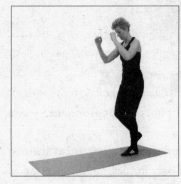
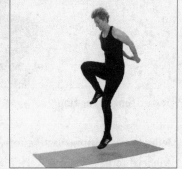

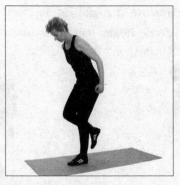

Lateral Single-Leg Hop

Medium-High Intensity: the lateral single-leg hop is particularly beneficial to basketball players, not only for developing lower-body explosive power but also in training the stabilisers of the hip and ankle, helping to protect the knees. This exercise will focus on a hop-stabilise sequence (not continuous).

Note: focus on exploding into the hop, then landing and stabilising without taking an extra step.

Instructions:
A. Set up from a loaded position, standing on your left leg.
B. Push off with the left foot with maximum power, using the right knee and arm swing to propel sideways and upwards. Keep your body straight.
C. Land on the sole (flatfooted) of the left foot and stabilise without taking any extra steps. Continue for prescribed hops and then repeat with opposite leg.

Exercise Target: reactive strength; develop vertical-jump power; develop ability to decelerate and stabilise under control.

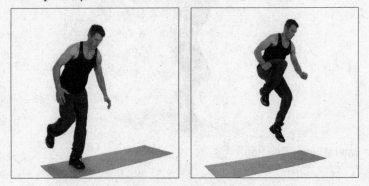

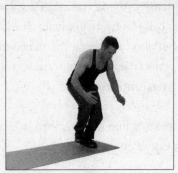

45-Degree Single-Leg Hop

Medium-High Intensity: the 45-degree single-leg hop is particularly beneficial to basketball and football (soccer) players, not only for developing lower-body explosive power but also in training the stabilisers of the hip and ankle, helping to protect the knees. This exercise will focus on a hop-stabilise sequence (not continuous).

Note: focus on exploding into the hop, then landing and stabilising without taking an extra step.

Instructions:

A. Set up from a loaded position, standing on your left leg.

B. Push off with the left foot with maximum power, using the right knee and arm swing to propel upwards and forwards at a 45° angle. Keep your body straight.

C. Land on the sole (flatfooted) of the left foot and stabilise without taking any extra steps. Continue for prescribed hops and then repeat with the opposite leg.

Exercise Target: reactive strength; develop vertical-jump power; develop ability to decelerate and stabilise under control.

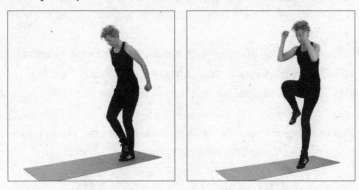

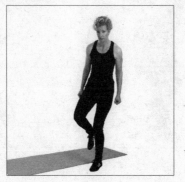

Forward-and-Back Single-Leg Hop

Medium-High Intensity: the forward-and-back single-leg hop is particularly beneficial to basketball and football players for developing lower-body explosive power, training the stabilisers of the hip and ankle and improving rapid-reaction motor skills.

Note: focus on speed with minimal floor-contact time.

Instructions:
A. Set up from a loaded position, standing on your left leg.
B. Push off with the left foot with maximum power, using the arms to assist momentum.
C. Land on the ball of the left foot. Reverse the movement by instantly pushing powerfully backwards into the start position. Continue for prescribed hops and then repeat with opposite leg.

Exercise Target: reactive strength; develop horizontal (plane) power; develop ability to rapidly change direction.

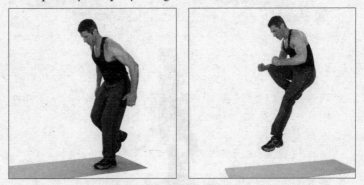

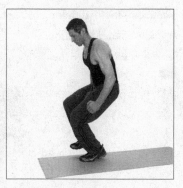

Side-to-Side Single-Leg Hop

Medium-High Intensity: the side-to-side single-leg hop is particularly beneficial to basketball and football players for developing lower-body explosive power, training the stabilisers of the hip and ankle and improving rapid-reaction motor skills.

Note: focus on speed with minimal floor-contact time.

Instructions:
A. Set up from a loaded position, standing on your left leg.
B. Push off with the left foot, jumping laterally with maximum power, using the arms to assist momentum.
C. Land on the ball of the left foot. Reverse the movement by instantly pushing powerfully back into the start position. Continue for prescribed hops and then repeat with opposite leg.

Exercise Target: reactive strength; develop horizontal (plane) power; develop ability to rapidly change direction.

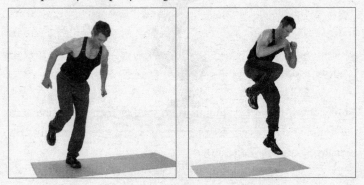

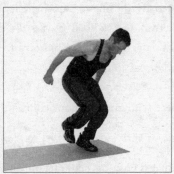

Standing Vertical Jump

Medium Intensity: the standing vertical jump is often used to assess an athlete's vertical-jump ability. This measurement is used to chart vertical jump-height progress and, in some instances, the data is used to assess anaerobic power and muscular endurance. Participants in basketball, football, rugby, volleyball and other sports involving vertical-jump elements will benefit from these plyometrics.

To chart your own vertical-jump progress, use this simple formula: stand on a flat, level surface next to a flat wall. Keeping your feet flat on the floor, extend your arm and mark off the highest point you can reach. Next, perform several standing vertical jumps and mark off the highest point. Finally, measure the distance between the two markers and you are left with your vertical-jump height. Use this figure in going forward to assess improvements. These can be performed as single repetitions or multiple continuous (higher intensity).

Note: concentrate on exploding as fast and as high as possible into the jump. Focus on counter-movements: rapid knee bend and arm swings prior to take off.

Instructions:
A. Start by standing in a neutral position.
B. Rapidly bend your knees, simultaneously bringing the arms back to create momentum.
C. Powerfully thrust your arms over your head as your legs extend. Reach as high as possible. Land softly. Repeat for prescribed repetitions and sets.

Exercise Target: reactive strength; develop vertical power.

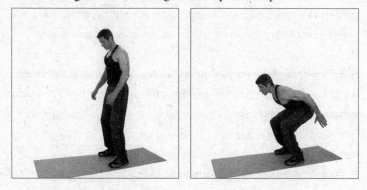

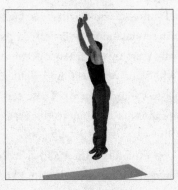

Box Jump

High Intensity: the box jump is a high-intensity plyometric. *Only perform this exercise if you can find a stable enough base.* It is included in the book as we have depth jumps performed off an elevation; however, a chair is not sufficient. (A flat-ledged wall or solid bench would work but take great care.)

These can be performed with a jump up/step down or continuously up and down for reps. Perform these *only* with the step-down version, as the continuous method exposes you to potential Achilles tendon tears. Only perform the jump up/jump down if you are preparing for competitive sport and, even then, approach with caution. This is a powerful movement with benefits in co-ordination and agility.

Note: concentrate on exploding as fast and as high as possible into the jump. Focus on counter-movements: rapid knee bend and arm swings prior to take off.

Instructions:
A. Position a box of appropriate height (elevation) approximately a foot in front of you. Stand with feet shoulder-width apart, with a

neutral spine, joints aligned and facing forward, arms by your sides.

B. Perform a semi-squat and rebound out of this position, extend through hips, knees and ankles and plantar-flex the feet. Jump as high as possible, using arm swing to assist.

C. Land on the elevation with knees bent to absorb the impact. Step down and repeat for repetitions. If when you land the knees 'cave in', bring the feet a little closer in the set-up.

Exercise Target: reactive strength; develop vertical power.

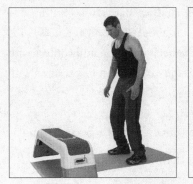
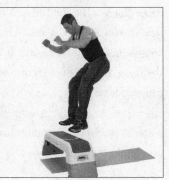

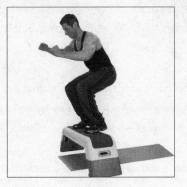

Depth Drop to Standing Long Jump

Ultra-High Intensity: this exercise is designed specifically to improve explosive sprinting power. The focus here is on rapid transition from landing to long jump. The conversion from vertical drop into horizontal plane reinforces the explosive forward momentum conducive to sprinting. The key here is to initiate minimal contact with the floor, landing only on the balls of the feet (no heel contact), then jumping as fast and as far as possible. The height of the drop dictates the load placed on landing; start lower and increase height over time (a regular chair is about 30cm off the floor, so is an adequate starting point). If the heels do come into contact with the floor, reduce the height until the exercise can be executed with proper form.

Note: concentrate on minimum contact with the ground; jump as fast and as far as possible.

Caution: this is an advanced plyometric. Only attempt it if you are accustomed to performing lower-intensity examples.

Instructions:

A. Start on an elevation (chair or step), standing in a neutral position.
B. Step off the elevation (do not jump) and drop to the floor, landing on the balls of both feet – with minimal flexion, absorb the shock with your ankles, knees and hips.
C. Use your arms for momentum and immediately explode into a forward jump.
D. Land on the soles of your feet (flatfooted) softly into a comfortable deep squat. Repeat for prescribed repetitions and sets.

Exercise Target: reactive strength; develop horizontal (plane) power.

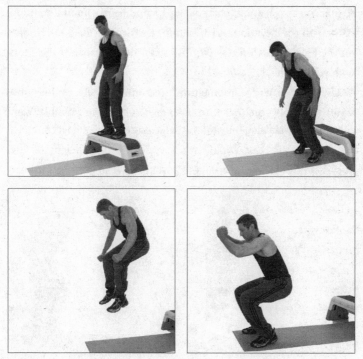

Depth Drop to Vertical Jump

Ultra-High Intensity: this exercise is designed specifically to improve jumping power and vertical-jump height, beneficial for basketball, football, rugby and other sports involving high-jump elements.

Note: concentrate on minimum contact with the ground; jump as fast and as high as possible.

Caution: this is an advanced plyometric. Only attempt it if you are accustomed to performing lower-intensity examples.

Instructions:

A. Start on an elevation (chair or step), standing in a neutral position.

B. Step off the elevation (do not jump) and drop to the floor, landing on the balls of both feet – with minimal flexion, absorb the shock with your ankles, knees and hips.

C. Use your arms for momentum and immediately explode into a vertical jump, reaching with both arms as high as possible. Land softly. Repeat for prescribed repetitions and sets.

Exercise Target: reactive strength; develop vertical jump power.

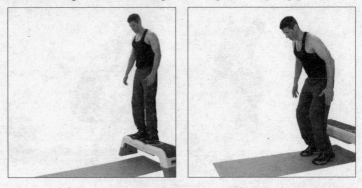

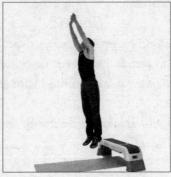

Multiple Standing Long Jumps

High Intensity: this exercise is designed specifically to improve sprinting power. The focus here is on rapid transition from jump to jump, maintaining forward momentum conducive to sprinting with minimum ground-contact time. Pay attention to co-ordinating arm swings with the lower body to produce forward drive. As these are multiple jumps, this exercise is best suited to outdoors (four to five jumps).

Note: concentrate on minimum contact with the ground and then jumping as fast and far as possible.

Caution: this is an advanced plyometric. Only attempt it if you are accustomed to performing lower-intensity examples.

Instructions:
A. Assume a standing long-jump position. Keep your chest over your knees and your knees over your feet.
B. Create momentum with the arms and explode forwards into the long jump.
C. Land on the balls of your feet.
D. Make a rapid transition into the next long jump by pushing off hard.

Exercise Target: reactive strength; develop horizontal (plane) power.

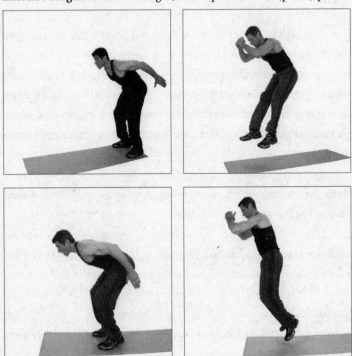

Forward Bounds

High Intensity: forward bounds are a classic sprinter's plyometric drill. The aim here is to mimic the sprinting stride, creating forward momentum with alternating pushes – force production framed within a sprint-specific movement pattern. This movement is quite technical so examine carefully before executing.

Note: concentrate on minimum contact with the ground and then jumping as fast and far as possible. Focus on quality, not quantity.

Caution: this is an advanced plyometric. Only attempt it if you are accustomed to performing lower-intensity examples.

Instructions:

A. Set up from a loaded position. Commit weight to your left leg and accentuate arm position. The rhythm of the movement is driven from the arms; pay attention to maintaining proper arm swing.

B. Push off with the left foot, driving off and out from the ground with maximum power. Bring the right leg forward, bending the knee until parallel with the ground, the left leg now fully extended behind. Keep arms in a consistent big swing. The body should be leaning forward at about 45°.

C. Hold this position, 'floating' before landing on the sole (flatfooted) of your right foot. Making minimal contact with the ground, push hard with the right foot, reversing the process, bringing the left knee up and extending the right leg. Your arms assist with propulsion and maintaining rhythm. Remember to maintain full glute-extension and front-knee flexion through each push. Perform four to five bounds, or as prescribed.

Exercise Target: reactive strength; develop horizontal (plane) power.

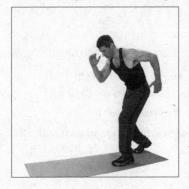 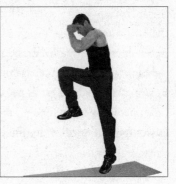

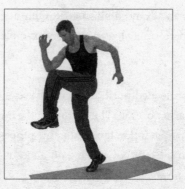

Hop, Skip and Jump

High Intensity: this plyometric drill teaches the body to change direction rapidly and powerfully – an essential component in almost all sports.

Note: concentrate on minimum contact with the ground and then jumping as fast and far as possible. Focus on transition from hop to skip to jump.

Caution: this is an advanced plyometric. Only attempt it if you are accustomed to performing lower-intensity examples.

Instructions:
A. Set up from a loaded position. Commit weight to slightly bent right leg with arms in preparatory position to assist propulsion.
B. Hop to the right as far as possible, landing on the right foot.
C. Immediately jump forward and land on the left foot.
D. Complete the drill with a final jump forward, landing on both feet.

Exercise Target: reactive strength; develop horizontal, vertical and directional power.

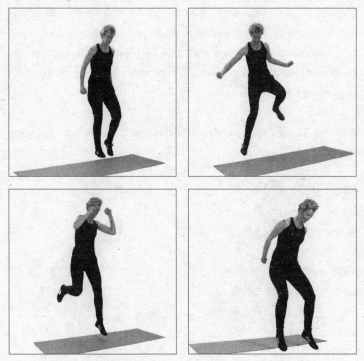

Kneeling Jump to Squat Hold

Ultra-High Intensity: this advanced plyometric drill requires considerable hip and glute activation – great benefits here for sprinters and jumpers.

Note: keeping the stretch cycle in mind, ensure you execute stage two quickly to generate momentum, using the arms also to great effect.
Caution: this is an advanced plyometric. Only attempt it if you are accustomed to performing lower-intensity examples.

Instructions:

A. Begin by kneeling on the floor, legs spread slightly wider than hips.

B. With a quick movement, sit back with your hips until your glutes touch your heels. Draw the arms back to generate momentum.

C. Forcefully use the arms and hips to bring the feet under the body and into a squat position. Return to the kneeling position for prescribed repetitions.

Exercise Target: reactive strength; develop horizontal and vertical power.

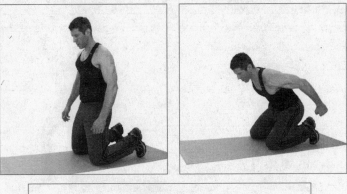

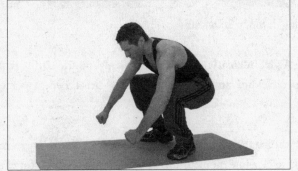

Horizontal Jump to Tuck Jump

High Intensity: the combination and transition of these two jumps teaches the body to quickly and powerfully change directions – useful for almost any sport.

Note: approach transitions as quickly as possible.
Caution: this is an advanced plyometric. Only attempt it if you are accustomed to performing lower-intensity examples.

Instructions:
A. Set up from a loaded position with feet together, knees slightly bent and arms drawn back to generate momentum.
B. Jump as far as possible horizontally.
C. Land on both feet, then immediately explode into a vertical 'tuck jump', drawing the knees into the chest.
D. Upon landing, jump in the opposite direction and repeat for prescribed repetitions.

Exercise Target: reactive strength; develop horizontal and vertical power.

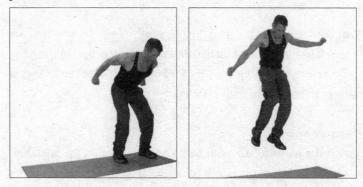

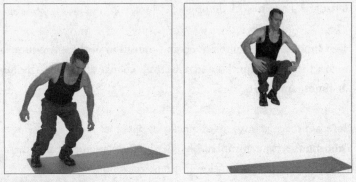

CORE EXERCISES

Crunch

The crunch is the most consummate *rectus abdominis* exercise. The short range of motion isolates the abdominals without assistance from the hip flexors (unlike the sit-up). Perform these with feet flat or, to increase the intensity, with feet elevated. However, it is prudent to note that, as popular as crunches are in the misguided concept of a 'six pack', their main function is to flex the spine (bending forwards). Our rectus-abdominis six pack, or even eight pack, lies beneath subcutaneous fat – *remove the fat and reveal the abs.*

Caution: use crunches sparingly, especially if you have lower-back issues. The range of motion dynamically reinforces the same inactive posture as when sitting at a desk for hours. The same can be said of sit-ups (not included in this book).

Instructions:
A. Lie flat on your back with bent knees, feet flat on the floor, hip-width apart. Hands can be placed in several different positions, either

crossed on your chest or beside or behind your head (if behind your head, do not use your hands to support or pull your head up).

B. Flex the abdominals, gently pulling them inwards, raising the torso up and lifting only the upper body off the floor. Keep your head in line with your spine. Hold for a second at the top of the movement and return the upper body to the floor. Perform prescribed repetitions.

Main Target: abs (rectus abdominis).

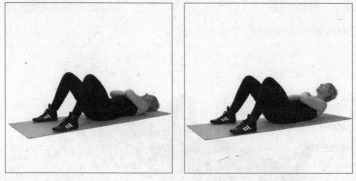

Alternate Crunch

This version of the crunch targets the obliques with assistance from the abs.

Caution: use alternate crunches sparingly, especially if you have lower-back issues. The range of motion dynamically reinforces the same inactive posture as when sitting at a desk for hours. The same can be said of sit-ups (not included in this book).

Instructions:

A. Lie flat on your back with the right leg flat and left knee bent. Place the hands beside the head.

B. Simultaneously raise the upper body, bringing the left elbow towards the right knee. Return the upper body to the floor and put the right leg flat. Repeat the process by again flexing and twisting the waist and flexing the hip and knee of the right leg. Perform prescribed repetitions.

C. Reverse for the opposite arm and leg by starting with the left leg flat and right knee bent. Flex and twist the waist, bringing the right elbow to meet the left knee. Perform prescribed repetitions.

Main Target: side of waist (obliques)

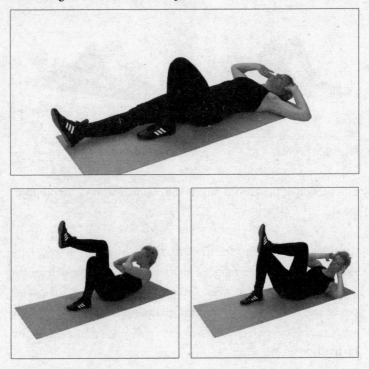

Seated Row Crunch

The seated row crunch is so named due to its rowing action. Perform this abdominal exercise by stabilising with the hands on the floor, or a more intense version with arms across the chest.

Instructions:
A. Sit on your backside with flexed knees drawn into your chest. Place your arms across the chest or hands on the floor to support (easier).
B. Fully extend the legs, simultaneously hinging backwards, then flex the knees and return to the start position. Perform prescribed repetitions.

Main Target: abs (rectus abdominis)

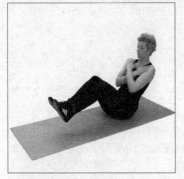 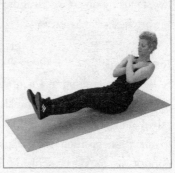

Seated Row-Crunch Hold

Isometric: the seated row-crunch isometric hold is the static version of the seated row-crunch exercise. Maintaining this position uses the inner abs to greater effect.

Instructions:

A. Sit on your backside with flexed knees drawn into chest. Place your arms across the chest or hands on the floor to support (easier).
B. Fully extend the legs, simultaneously hinging backwards. Hold this position for the prescribed time period.

Main Target: abs (rectus abdominis) and inner abs (transverse abdominis)

Single-Leg Hold

Isometric: the single-leg hold conditions the core muscles in stabilising. Use your arms to assist in balance, or increase the intensity by holding them across your chest. Pay attention to keeping the leg low, focusing on core activation; raising the leg higher will bring in the hip flexors to assist.

Instructions:

A. Begin by standing in a neutral position. Commit weight to your left foot, brace your abdominals (including inner units) and then raise your right foot a few inches off the floor. Keep the core engaged to maintain position for the prescribed time. Alternate with the opposite leg for the prescribed time.

Main Target: abs (rectus abdominis) and inner abs (transverse abdominis)

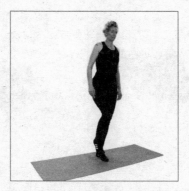

Oblique Crunch

This specifically targets the external and internal obliques. Pay special attention to execution.

Instructions:

A. Lie on your left side, resting on your left arm with knees together and legs bent (at approximately 20°).

B. Squeeze your oblique, raising your legs off the floor and bringing them towards your chest at a 45° angle. Simultaneously bring the torso towards the knees. Reverse the action and complete for prescribed reps, then alternate.

Main Target: side of waist (internal and external obliques).

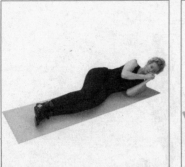 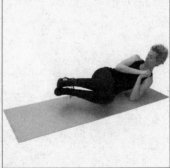

Reverse Curl

This activates the transverse abdominis and helps recruit pelvic floor muscles – an essential component to any complete core-strengthening program and included throughout this book.

Instructions:

A. Lie flat on your back, placing your hands behind (or if you have neck issues, in front of) your head, knees bent and feet crossed.

B. Keep your head on the floor and bring your knees towards your chest, rounding your lower back and lifting your backside off the floor. As well as working the TrA, the pelvic floor is engaged when drawing the knees up. This should be a smooth, short range of motion.

Main Target: inner abs (transverse abdominis)

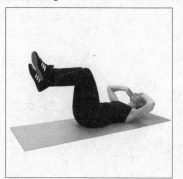 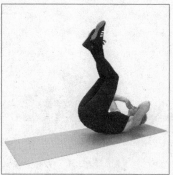

Bicycle

To gain the full benefits with this exercise, perform rotations with a slow cadence.

Instructions:

A. Assume the start position by lying on your back and placing your fingers on your temples, lifting your upper back slightly off the floor. Engage your abs and bring the right knee towards the chest. Simultaneously extend the left leg (keep above hip height). Rotate the torso, bringing the left elbow towards the right knee.

B. Slowly exchange leg and elbow positions so that the right elbow is brought towards the left knee while the right leg goes into extension. Perform these cycling rotations with a slight pause – count to two before alternating.

Main Target: abs (abdominis rectus)

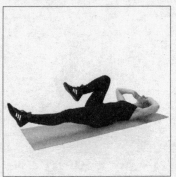 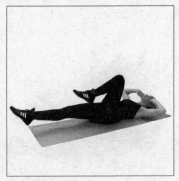

Russian Twist

To gain the full benefits with this exercise, perform rotations with a slow cadence. Keep the inner abs contracted throughout the rotations.

Instructions:

A. Assume the start position by sitting on your backside. Bend the knees and bring the legs together. Brace the abs and lift the legs off the floor, position the arms in front with fingers interlaced.

B. Rotate the trunk from side to side, keeping your head in line with your spine. Perform in a smooth motion for prescribed repetitions.

Main Target: abs (abdominis rectus), side/front of waist (internal and external obliques), inner abs (transverse abdominis)

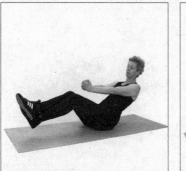 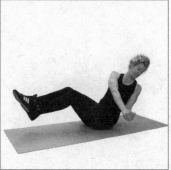

Climbing Twist

The climbing twist develops both internal and external units of the core, improving stability and movement initiation.

Instructions:

A. Assume the start position of the standard press-up, hands shoulder-width apart, in a straight line from head to heel with feet hip-width apart, abs braced (core engaged).

B. Rotate the trunk, drawing the left knee towards the right elbow and return to the start position. Alternate with the right knee to the left elbow. Continue to alternate for the prescribed repetitions.

Main Target: side/front of waist (internal and external obliques), inner abs (transverse abdominis), abs (abdominis rectus).

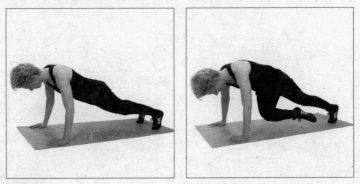

Bird Dog

The bird dog focuses on the lower back. Keep the action smooth and non-jerky, taking both limbs to full extension and back.

Instructions:

A. Assume a quadrupedal position (on all fours, hands directly below shoulders and knees hip-width apart), head in line with spine and flat back.

B. Simultaneously extend the left arm in front and right leg behind in one smooth movement until both limbs are fully extended. Return to starting position and repeat for prescribed repetitions. Once completed, reverse to the opposite hand and leg and repeat.

Main Target: lower back (erector spinae).

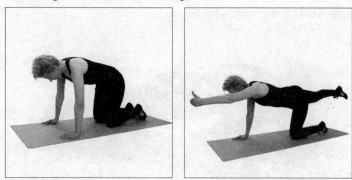

Plank

Isometric: the plank is an isometric exercise included in this section as it targets the abs. Pay special attention here not to let the hips sag and put strain through your lower back. The exercise focus is to keep the body prone and abs engaged throughout the allotted timeframe.

Caution: although useful, the plank creates a compressing effect on the spine that could potentially exacerbate any existing lower-back condition.

Instructions:

A. Assume a prone position on your elbows (in line with your shoulders), feet together or hip-width apart. Activate the abdominals to maintain the prone position without letting the hips sag and keep a straight line from head to heel. Keep the abs contracted for the required timescale; then relax.

Main Target: abs (rectus abdominis), lower back (erector spinae), inner abs (transverse abdominis).

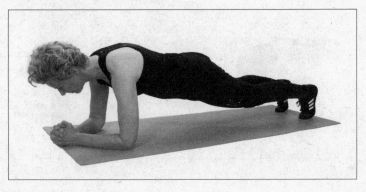

Plank with Raised Leg

This is a more challenging core isometric than the standard plank. The raised leg engages the lower back and contributes to further benefits in stabilisation.

Caution: although useful, the plank creates a compressing effect on the spine that could potentially exacerbate any existing lower-back condition.

Instructions:

Assume a prone position on your elbows (in line with your shoulders), feet together or hip-width apart. Activate the abdominals to maintain the prone position without letting the hips sag and keeping a straight line from head to heel. Lift one leg off the floor and hold this position for a time before returning and repeating with the opposite leg.

Main Target: abs (rectus abdominis), lower back (erector spinae), inner abs (transverse abdominis).

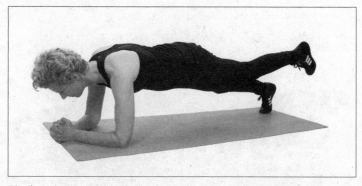

Plank with Lateral Shift

This incorporates movement into the standard plank. Pay special attention here not to let the hips sag, putting strain through your lower back. The exercise focus is to keep the body prone and the core engaged while shifting foot position from side to side.

Caution: although useful, the plank creates a compressing effect on the spine that could potentially exacerbate any existing lower-back condition. Focus must be kept on keeping the transverse abdominis fully engaged throughout.

Instructions:

A. Assume a prone position on your elbows (in line with your shoulders), feet together or hip-width apart. Activate the abdominals to maintain the prone position without letting the hips sag and keeping a straight line from head to heel.

B. From this position, step the left foot out and back in, then repeat with the right foot. Continue to alternate for prescribed repetitions.

Main Target: abs (rectus abdominis), lower back (erector spinae) and inner abs (transverse abdominis).

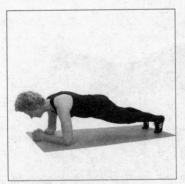
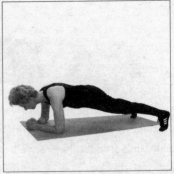

Side Plank

This is another isometric exercise included in the core section as it targets the obliques (side of waist, outer and inner). Variations of this exercise are side plank with a twist and side plank repetitions.

Instructions:

Lie on your side with legs positioned one on top of the other and body supported on your elbow with arm straight. Raise the body off the floor by contracting the oblique to maintain a straight line from elbow to heel. Keep the body rigid for the prescribed time period; then repeat on the opposite side.

Main Target: side of waist (internal and external obliques), inner abs (transverse abdominis), hip (adductor muscles of the hip).

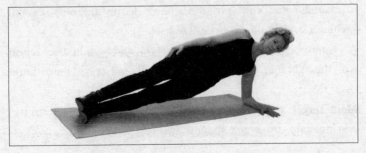

Side Plank with Twist

This adds a further dimension to the side plank.

Instructions:

A. Lie on your side with legs positioned one on top of the other and body supported on your elbow with arm straight. Raise the body off the floor by contracting the oblique and laterally flexing the spine to maintain a straight line from elbow to heel.

B. From this position, twist from the waist, bringing the elbow towards the floor, then unfurl back to the starting position, keeping the oblique contracted throughout. Perform prescribed repetitions then repeat with the opposite side.

Main Target: side of waist (internal and external obliques), inner abs (transverse abdominis), hip (adductor muscles of the hip)

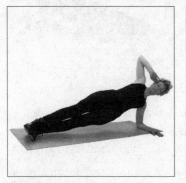 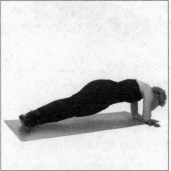

Side Plank for Reps

This converts the isometric standard plank into a dynamic repetition-based exercise.

Instructions:

A. Lie on your side with legs positioned one on top of the other, the body supported on your elbow with arm straight. Raise the body off the floor by contracting the oblique and laterally flexing the spine to maintain a straight line from elbow to heel.

B. Let the hips drop to the floor, then contract the oblique and flex the spine once again – that's one rep. Repeat in smooth movements, then perform on the opposite side.

Main Target: side of waist (internal and external obliques), inner abs (transverse abdominis), hip (adductor muscles of the hip)

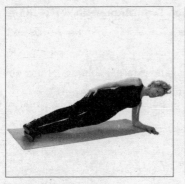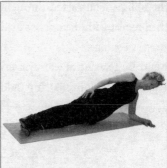

Superman/Alternate

The Superman focuses on the lower back. This can also be performed alternating the opposite arm to leg (left arm and right leg raised simultaneously, then right arm and left leg – continue to alternate). Keep this action very smooth and controlled with no jerky movements.

Instructions:

A. Lie on your front with your arms extended.

B. Simultaneously raise your arms and legs off the floor. Keep a smooth action throughout. Repeat for prescribed repetitions.

Main Target: lower back (erector spinae).

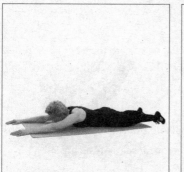 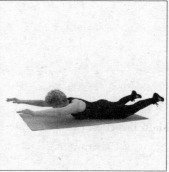

V-UP

This targets the abdominals but also conditions the hip flexors and improves balance. The V-UP and alternate V-UP are the only two double-leg lifts included in this book.

Caution: if you have a bad lower back, this exercise compresses the lumbar segments (lower spine). The force generated from lifting the legs causes the hip flexors to pull on the lumbar vertebrae. Having said this, some find this exercise very beneficial and retain it within their program (hence I've included it here). If you are going to use it, *ensure you 'round out' your lower spine to protect against injury*.

Instructions:
A. Lie flat on your back, arms extended above your head.
B. Contract the abs and raise the trunk, simultaneously bringing the legs and hands together to form a V-shape. Return to the start position under control, ensuring your upper back touches down. Keep legs straight throughout; avoid jerking them, to protect the spine. Perform prescribed repetitions.

Main Target: abs (rectus abdominis)

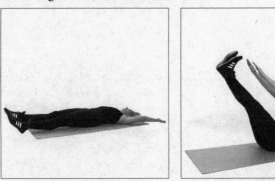

V-UP Alternate

This targets the abdominals but also conditions the hip flexors and improves balance. The V-UP and alternate V-UP are the only two double-leg lifts included in this book.

Caution: if you have a bad lower back, this exercise compresses the lumbar segments (lower spine). The force generated from lifting the legs causes the hip flexors to pull on the lumbar vertebrae. Having said this, some find this exercise very beneficial and retain it within their program (hence I've included it here). If you are going to use it, *ensure you 'round out' your lower spine to protect against injury.*

Instructions:
A. Lie flat on your back, arms extended above your head.
B. Contract the abs and raise the trunk, simultaneously bringing the left leg and right hand together to form a V-shape. Return to the start position under control, ensuring your upper back touches down. Alternate with opposite leg to opposite hand. Keep legs straight throughout; avoid jerking them, to protect the spine. Perform prescribed repetitions.

Main Target: abs (rectus abdominis).

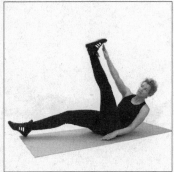

Jack-Knife Sit-Up

This is a powerful abdominal exercise involving co-ordination and balance.

Caution: those with lower-back issues may want to reconsider this exercise.

Instructions:

A. Lie flat on your back, arms by your sides.

B. Contract the abs, bringing the trunk and knees together. Extend the hips and knees back to the start position and perform prescribed repetitions.

Main Target: abs (rectus abdominis)

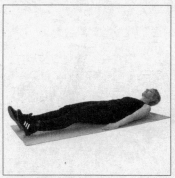
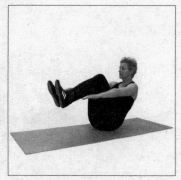

Leg Passes

These target the transverse abdominis, the deepest and subtlest of the abdominal muscles. This often-neglected muscle plays a critical role in stabilising the spine and pelvis; by strengthening it, you not only benefit your overall core strength but also prevent potential back injury.

Instructions:

A. Begin by lying flat on your back, arms extended above your head, knees bent and feet flat on the floor.

B. Bring the right knee towards the chest as far as possible. As you return the leg to the floor, bring the left leg simultaneously towards the chest so that they *pass* in mid-air.

C. Continue this cycling action with bent knees (do not straighten the legs; let the heels just brush the floor as they return). With correct execution, the abdomen should be flat or hollowed.

Main Target: inner abs (transverse abdominis).

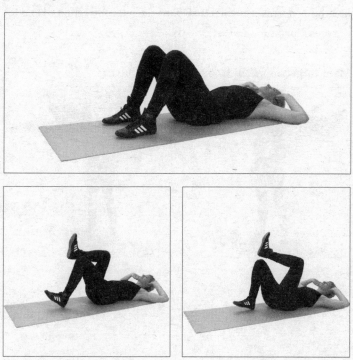

Vacuum

The vacuum is an isometric exercise included here as it targets the TrA, the deepest and most difficult to reach of the abdominal muscles. This often-neglected muscle plays a critical role in stabilising the spine and pelvis; by strengthening it you not only benefit your overall core strength but also prevent potential back injury.

Instructions:

A. Stand in a neutral position with your feet shoulder-width apart.

B. Inhale, fully raising the rib cage. Exhale, keeping your rib cage elevated and bringing your belly button towards your spine. Visualise retracting as far back to your spine as possible. During the contraction, breathe as normal (it will feel shallow during contraction). Hold for the prescribed time and sets.

Main Target: inner abs (transverse abdominis).

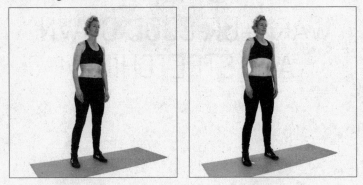

CHAPTER SEVEN

WARM-UP, COOL-DOWN AND STRETCHING

Preparing the body for exercise (warm-up), returning it to a pre-exercise state (cool-down) and maintaining and developing range of motion (post-exercise stretching) are all-important factors in maintaining mobility, flexibility and preventing injury. I will keep this relatively brief, as I am sure you already have a procedure in place!

The warm-up here is a general one. Depending on the rapid-workout you select, your warm-up might be more workout-specific – e.g. if the workout is plyometric, you would factor in more dynamic stretches (explained later on) that simulate (at a low intensity) the ensuing high-intensity movements.

Warm-up explained

To optimise performance it is advisable to warm up prior to exercise and allow the body make the necessary adjustments in breathing, heart rate and blood flow. This is a gradual process and should be approached with a steady increase in intensity. Entering into a strenuous workout without an appropriate warm-up could result in injury.

The main benefits to the warm-up are:

- reduced muscle stiffness (using dynamic stretching), considered a main factor in muscle injury;
- increased temperature and blood flow to muscles and enhanced delivery of oxygen;
- vital organs reaching a workable rate for the level of exercise;
- mobilisation of joints and warming of synovial fluid (which nourishes, lubricates and shock-absorbs synovial joints: elbow, shoulder, hip, knee, etc);
- preparation of neuromuscular pathways and motor units for subsequent exercise;
- mental preparation for subsequent exercise.

Recent research has suggested that dynamic stretching (slow, controlled movements through full ROM) is more beneficial during the warm-up than static stretching (static holds). Observation suggested dynamic stretching was more effective at reducing muscle stiffness (the main factor in muscle injury) than its counterpart. Conversely, static stretching is *more* beneficial post-workout due to its relaxing effect on the muscles and facilitating increased ROM. There has been much conjecture as regards the appropriate pre-exercise procedure – if you have always statically stretched prior to your workouts and it works for you, continue. The science behind warming-up is not conclusive. However, the dynamic approach has always seemed logical to me, as the mimicking of subsequent movements gradually prepares the body for what's to come; relaxing the muscle with static stretching would appear to be counter-productive and may potentially expose you to injury.

Warm-up exercises

1. Begin with walking on the spot and gradually take it up into a light jog for three to four minutes. You could also use a gentle version of boxing uppercuts or straights (p.107-9).
2. Perform mobilising exercises to articulate the joints.
3. Perform dynamic stretching exercises; choose those that more closely mimic the workout you are going to perform (e.g. gentle squats, lunges and calf raises if your workout is lower-body plyometric).

The total time for your warm-up should be between five and ten minutes; this is very much specific to your personal needs (you may have areas that warrant particular attention in terms of warming up). Also, your starting preparedness will depend on how warm you are to begin with (i.e. on the climate).

Mobilising and dynamic stretching

Start by mobilising the joints with small rotations and work up towards larger dynamic stretching movements, standing in an upright position with neutral spine.

Rotating approximately five times clockwise and five times anti-clockwise is sufficient. Maintain smooth and rhythmical movements.

Wrists: gently circle.
Ankles: commit weight to one leg, raise the ankle and circle gently.
Head: rotate head left and right, then back and forth smoothly.

Shoulder rolls: keeping arms bent, smoothly roll the shoulders forwards then backwards.

Trunk rotation: with arms held in front of you, rotate the trunk, keeping your lower-body fixed, to the left and right in a smooth, gentle action.

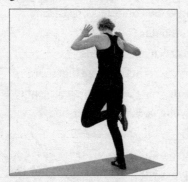

Side bends: gently reach down to the side, alternating for five reps on each side.

Hip circles: circle the hips both clockwise and anti-clockwise.

Arm swings: swing both arms clockwise and anti-clockwise.

Flick-backs: stand with feet shoulder-width apart, then alternate flicking your heel towards your backside, transferring weight to the supporting foot as you go. Repeat alternately for five reps per side.

Elbow to knee trunk twist: bring your knee to the opposite elbow. Repeat alternately for five reps per side.

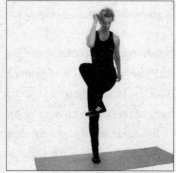

Alternate lunge: follow the instructions on page 73 of the Exercise Portfolio. Repeat alternately for five reps per leg.

Side lunge: follow the instructions on page 75 of the Exercise Portfolio. Repeat alternately for five reps per leg.

Squats: follow the instructions on page 66 of the Exercise Portfolio. Perform six to eight reps.

Butt kicks: increase the intensity with butt kicks. Jog on the spot, keeping your arms by your side, bringing your heels towards your backside.

Leg swings: use a wall or solid base to stabilise. Commit weight to one leg and swing forward and backwards. Perform six to eight reps on one leg and repeat with the opposite leg. The action should be controlled and smooth.

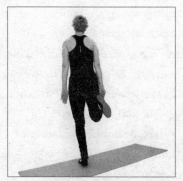

This list is simply a general approach to the warm-up. You might want to add or remove certain exercises or place more emphasis on particular areas. Whatever your approach, you should definitely warm up!

Cool-down and post-workout static stretching explained

This is often a neglected component of a workout but, to ensure longevity, this post-workout procedure is important and must be included to achieve holistic benefits.

We cool down to:
- gradually return the heart rate and breathing to resting levels (abrupt cessation of exercise can be harmful for the heart);
- gently return blood flow to a pre-exercise state, avoiding blood pooling in the leg muscles that could lead to dizziness or fainting;
- remove waste products (e.g. lactic acid), effectively removed by gentle exercise.

Cool down for several minutes, using a rhythmical exercise similar to warming up: light jogging on the spot or a gentle version of boxing uppercuts/straights from the Exercise Portfolio (p.107).

Static stretching

As mentioned previously, static stretching is most effective post-exercise. The muscles are still warm and pliable and contain more blood, so offer greater protection against injury.

The aim here is to:
- relax the muscles and restore them to their resting length, improving flexibility and mobility (ROM);
- remove waste products;
- prepare the muscles for the next workout;
- potentially prevent delayed-onset muscle soreness (DOMS), the post-workout discomfort usually associated with unfamiliar exercise or increases in intensity. The evidence that stretching prevents DOMS is inconclusive; nevertheless, it has other benefits which should not be ignored.

There are two types of approaches with post-workout stretches: 'maintenance' and 'developmental'.

Maintenance stretches are held for approximately 10–15 seconds at the 'bite' (when the pull is felt). This stretch will lengthen the muscle, maintain flexibility and prevent muscle soreness.

Developmental stretches are held for 25–30 seconds at the bite until the tension eases, at which point the muscle is externally stretched further to increase length and ROM.

Ensure you breathe while stretching, remembering that this helps to relax the blood flow throughout the body and assists the removal of waste products.

STRETCHES

Perform these for the desired time between ten and thirty seconds, depending on the stretch target: 'maintenance' or 'developmental'.

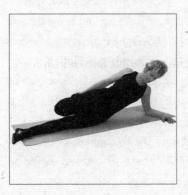

Lying upper leg: quadriceps and patellar tendon stretch

1. Lie on your side.
2. Pull the heel towards the backside until you feel a pull or 'bite' on your thigh and knee. Hold the stretch for the desired time.
3. Repeat with opposite leg.

Standing posterior upper thigh: hamstring stretch

1. From a standing position, extend your left leg in front, resting on the heel of your foot.
2. Place your hands and weight onto your right leg, keeping the back flat and sitting back into the stretch. The more you sit back, the more intense the pull on the hamstring. Hold the stretch for the desired time.
3. Repeat with opposite leg.

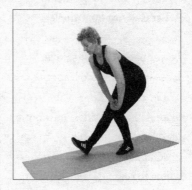

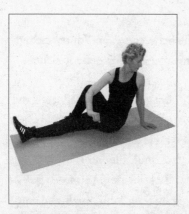

Upper and lower back: erector spinae, latissimus dorsi and trapezius

1. Sitting on the floor, extend your right leg and bring the left leg over the right, resting the left foot outside the right knee.

2. Rest the right elbow on the outside of the left thigh, placing the left arm behind.

3. Rotate the torso towards the left arm. Use the right elbow to apply pressure to the left knee, furthering the stretch. The stretch should be felt in the lower back (also, in some instances, on the outside of your left leg). Hold the stretch for the desired time.

4. Repeat with opposite leg.

Lower back: erector spinae, latissimus dorsi and trapezius

1. Lie on the floor, with arms extended either side. Draw both legs together, feet flat.

2. Keeping the knees together, rotate to one side under smooth control and hold the stretch through the lower back. Keep

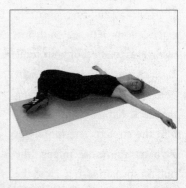

the shoulders on the floor throughout. Hold for the desired time, then gently reverse and rotate to the other side.

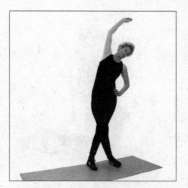

Outer thigh: iliotibial band (ITB)

1. From a standing position, cross your right foot behind your left foot so your feet are parallel.

2. Lean to the left and shift your weight onto your right leg, pushing your right hip outwards. With correct application, the stretch should be felt in your right hip and along the outside of your thigh. Hold the stretch for the desired time.

3. Repeat with opposite leg.

Backside/glutes: gluteus maxi-mus and piriformis

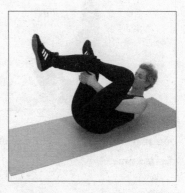

1. Begin by lying on your back. Draw your knees towards your chest, placing your left ankle over your right knee.

2. Next, reach under your right thigh; the left arm goes through the gap in the bent leg and the right arm around the side. With the correct application, the stretch should be felt in the gluteal region. Hold the stretch for the desired time.

3. Repeat with opposite leg.

Pelvis: Hip flexors and iliopsoas

1. Start from a standing neutral position, hands on hips.

2. Take a comfortable step forward into a lunge position, keeping the torso upright. The stretch will be felt in the 'open' hip. Hold the stretch for the desired time.

2. Repeat with the opposite leg.

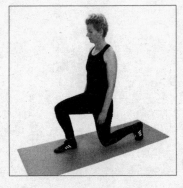

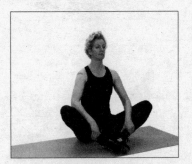

Inner thigh/groin muscles: adductors

1. Start from a seated position, back upright with the soles of your feet together.

2. Apply pressure with the elbows, until stretch is felt in the upper groin (adductors).

You may be able to achieve this unassisted. Hold the stretch for the desired time.

Calf: gastrocnemius

1. Lean forward against a wall.

2. Bend the front leg and extend the back straight behind, keeping the heel on the floor. The stretch will be felt in the calf muscle. Increase the stretch by extending the leg further behind. Hold the stretch for the desired time.

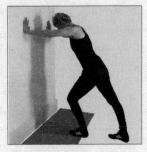

3. Repeat with the opposite leg.

Calf (outer): soleus

1. Lean forward against a wall.
2. Assume the same position as the gastrocnemius stretch, but this time bend the extended leg into the same position as the front leg. The stretch will be felt on the outside of the calf muscle. Hold the stretch for the desired time.
3. Repeat with the opposite leg.

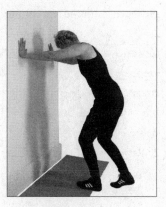

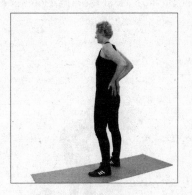

Chest: pectorals

1. Start from a standing position, placing the palms of your hands on your lower back.
2. Draw the elbows together until you feel a stretch across your chest. Hold the stretch for the desired time.

Shoulders: deltoids

1. Start from a standing position, drawing one arm across your chest.
2. Placing the opposite hand above the elbow (not *on* the elbow), apply pressure, drawing the elbow

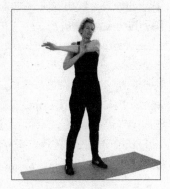

towards the chest. The stretch will be felt on the outside of the shoulder. Hold for the desired time.

3. Repeat with the opposite arm.

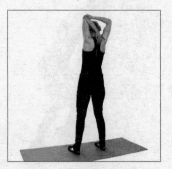

Back of arms: triceps

1. Start from a standing position. Bring one hand behind the head, drawing the hand towards the middle of the back, elbow pointing upwards.

2. Using the other hand, grasp the elbow and gently draw it towards the head. The stretch will be felt along the back of the arm. Hold for the desired time.

1. Repeat with the opposite arm.

Front of arms: biceps

1. Start from a standing position. Extend both arms behind you.

2. With palms facing upwards, draw the arms up to feel the stretch across both biceps. Hold for the desired time.

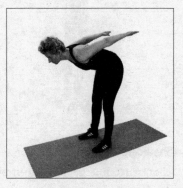

Nutrition

Needless to say, any successful fitness/training program should be accompanied by adequate nutrition; failure to implement good dietary practice will negatively affect performance levels, hinder progress and lead to physical breakdown. Sustenance is the most important aspect to a fitness program – afford it the same level of consideration as you do your workout for maximum benefit. There is a plethora of information on sports nutrition out there. Find and implement what complements your needs.

Considerations

If you are an athlete requiring muscle mass (rugby/American football) or a recreational exerciser in search of muscle growth (hypertrophy), you will want to consider factoring in more bodyweight-resistance workouts (rep range eight to twelve) and yielding isometrics (30–60-second holds). Alternatively, if it's maximal strength you want to develop, adaptations will be specific to an individual's current strength in relation to the exercise concerned. Naturally, there are many bodyweight exercises that could develop maximal strength that would represent an enormous challenge to *anyone* (such as gymnastics), but these are not included in this book as they represent very advanced propositions. Instead, select resistance exercises that represent the most challenging variation and work with these.

Improve your speed-strength/power with plyometrics, isometrics and complex training. It is important to remember that we can be strong and not powerful or, alternatively, fast and not strong. I propose for all athletes, whether recreational, amateur or professional, the inclusion of speed-strength/power workouts, as developing this area is critical to the majority of sports: football, rugby, tennis, boxing, weightlifting, hockey, basketball, netball, baseball, track and field all involve, to a greater or lesser degree, throwing, kicking, jumping, punching, sprinting, pushing, hopping, spinning, leaping and bounding. If you decide to use the rapid-workouts as a complete program, factor in adequate rest periods, and consider frequency and overall cycling of workouts.

Plyometric, isometric and complex training can be very taxing on the central nervous system (CNS), which, unlike muscular fatigue, can be difficult to identify and take much longer to present itself. The body needs time to replenish its energy stores and repair itself from the rigours of training and changing workout stimuli. Below are some general guidelines to consider when putting a program together.

General guidelines for usage

Isometric: general guidelines say no more than three to four times per week with no more than ten minutes total contraction time. Six-to-ten-second holds. Four to five weeks on, then layoff. Allow for CNS to recover. Two sessions is more than sufficient per week.

Plyometric: two to three sessions per week. Allow three days between sessions to recover. (These sessions do not include GPP, where low-intensity plyometrics are used, referring only to the individual plyometric workouts.) Those new to plyometric exercise should begin with 60–80 contacts per session and work up to 150–200 when more experienced. Four to five weeks on, then layoff. Allow for CNS to recover.

Tabata: one to two sessions per week. Four to five weeks, then layoff.

GPP: one to two sessions per week. Four to five weeks, then layoff.

Resistance: Two to three sessions per week, with 48 hours between each body part (if isolating). Cycle training through the strength continuum: four to five weeks strength; four to five weeks hypertrophy; four to five weeks endurance. This, of course, is personal to your requirements, but cycling in this way allows for CNS to recover and encourage further adaptations to new stimuli. It will manifest better long-term gains.

Recap

Obviously, if you are training for a specific event, you will have phases to adhere to, so pick and use the workouts which best complement your particular stage of training. As with recreational exercisers and sportspeople, decide what it is you actually want to achieve. Do you want to add more power to your vertical jumping ability? Or sprint faster by increasing your horizontal-plane power with forward bounds or multiple standing long jumps? You might want to pack on more muscle with resistance and isometric-resistance workouts? It may be you want to focus on the weaker aspects of your performance? Identify these and tailor your routine according. Be sensible, consider balance and be creative.

SAMPLE PROGRAMS

For those intending to use the rapid-workouts as a standalone program, I've created four different sample programs, three with individual training targets (speed strength, hypertrophy and endurance) and a fourth hybrid program combining all of the above. There are infinite ways you could use these workouts as a standalone program. I've included an AM and PM workout approach but you could collapse both sessions into one (as the workouts are short), taking an adequate rest between disciplines. Where the core is included, perform it as the last element. In addition, when selecting a workout from within a section (e.g. Tabata), choose the most suitable level of difficulty (you may find your level to be higher for some workouts and lower in others). You may just want to do one rapid-workout per day. If so, ensure you give it 100 per cent. When creating a bespoke program, stick to the principles in the book to understand why you are including a workout and for what benefit – tailor a combination that will propel your abilities to greater heights.

After four to five weeks, take a break from the high-intensity elements and continue with resistance workouts and more moderate exercise to recover. Return to high intensity after a month or so and continue the cycle.

Speed Strength / Power Development

Time	Mon	Tues	Weds	Thurs	Friday	Sat	Sun
AM	Overcoming Isometric & Core	Off	Complex Sets & Core	Tabata & Core	Off	Resistance Circuit & Core	Off
PM	Plyometric	Off	Off	Overcoming Isometric	Off	Plyometric	Off

Hypertrophy / Muscle-growth Development

Time	Mon	Tues	Weds	Thurs	Friday	Sat	Sun
AM	Tabata & Core	Off	Resistance Circuit & Core	Off	GPP & Core	Complex Sets & Core	Off
PM	Resistance Circuit	Off	Yielding Isometric	Off	Resistance Circuit	Off	Off

Muscle-endurance Development

Time	Mon	Tues	Weds	Thurs	Friday	Sat	Sun
AM	GPP & Core	Tabata & Core	Off	Tabata & Core	Off	GPP & Core	Off
PM	Off	Resistance Circuit (High rep)	Off	Resistance Circuit (High rep)	Off	Yielding Isometric	Off

Hybrid Development

Time	Mon	Tues	Weds	Thurs	Friday	Sat	Sun
AM	GPP & Core	Tabata & Core	Plyometric	GPP & Core	Resistance Circuit	Complex Set & Core	Off
PM	Resistance Circuit	Off	Yielding Isometric	Off	Overcoming Isometric	Off	Off

Remember to:

- wear the appropriate clothing, footwear, etc;
- ensure that your workout environment is clear of obstacles and, if performing plyometric exercises, that you have adequate headspace to perform jumps safely;
- warm up! Fail to do this to your detriment, as explained in the warm-up chapter;
- differentiate between exercise discomfort and pain – any sort of pain means you should desist immediately; continuing will exacerbate your condition and may result in medical complications;
- breathe! It's so often neglected, so exhale on the effort, as you push, pull or jump;
- focus on the workout at hand; be 'in the moment'; execute the workouts as described to achieve optimum results and avoid injury.

• pay special attention to mobilising the joints specific to the ensuing workout when performing plyometrics. (A thorough warm-up is essential, as with all the rapid-workouts.) The best surfaces for plyometrics would be grass or synthetic – concrete is not recommended. Good quality footwear with a cushioned sole is also advisable.

TABATA WORKOUTS

Read more on Tabata Workouts on page 21.

Guide

There are a variety of Tabata rapid-workouts in this section. 'Classic Tabata' should be approached faithfully, as detailed below. In addition, I have created 'Alternate Tabata' and 'Multi-Tabata' using the same regimen of 20 seconds work and 10 seconds rest. These will still be classified as HIIT. However, due to the increased volume of work, the intensity will be sub-maximal (RPE 6-7), seeing considerable benefits to muscular endurance. Factor these in with the Classic Tabata, keeping your workouts fresh and energised.

Frequency: one to two times per week (dependent on other HIIT workouts in a given week).

Equipment

A stopwatch is required as these are timed workouts. There are several free Apps available designed specifically for Tabata. I recommend a (currently) free timer called 'Tabata Timer' for the iPhone, designed by Garaio Technology Lab. Alternatively, for Android, download the (currently) free 'My Tabata Timer', designed by Ellerynz.

Approach

The Classic Tabata workouts should be approached with maximal intensity (RPE maximal) to enjoy the full benefits of the regimen. However, one can still benefit by starting at a sub-maximal level and working towards a higher intensity.

Use the Rate of Perceived Exertion Chart below to measure your intensity level.

Workout difficulty level

Each workout has a 'workout difficulty' number: the higher the number, the more challenging the workout. Note that exercise selection is key with Tabata, as the exercise must present a significant enough challenge to perform eight sets at maximal intensity but, at the same time, not be overly strenuous. If you are new to Tabata, begin with workout-difficulty level one and work your way up. Be creative and experiment, using alternative exercises from the Exercise Portfolio.

Borg CR10 Scale

Intensity / Effort	
0	No exertion at all
0.5	Extremely light
1	Very light
2	Fairly light
3	Moderate
4	Somewhat hard
5	Hard
6	
7	Very hard
8	
9	
10	Extremely hard
*	Maximal Tabata Zone

Caution: these programs are not suitable for beginners – a solid fitness background is required before taking part. If you are untrained, sedentary, have underlying health problems or biomechanical issues, it is inadvisable to participate at this level of activity, as there is an increased risk of injury. If in doubt, seek medical advice before attempting any of the workouts.

HIIT/CLASSIC TABATA REGIMEN
Workout 1
Develop: anaerobic threshold, VO2max capacity, fast-twitch fibres and increase EPOC effect.
Workout difficulty: 1

Exercise	Sets	Work Intervals	Rest Intervals	Intensity	Total time
Jumping Jack	8	20 Sec	10 Sec	Ultra-High	4 Minutes

When using as a standalone workout, include warm-up (five-to-ten minutes), cool-down and stretch (four-to-five minutes). Warm-up time will be specific to your requirements and conditions. Cool down and stretching time varies and depends on the stretch focus (maintenance or development). Read more on warm-up p.173, cool-down and stretching p.177. Alternatively, filter this workout directly into your existing program (with the assumption that you have already warmed up).

Visual exercise reference

Warm-up exercises   175
Jumping Jack   110

Exercise Guide Note: the Tabata workout consists of 8 x 20-second intervals interspersed with 10-second rest periods. Each interval should be approached with maximum intensity (see RPE chart). Use the rest periods to recover as much as possible before exploding into the next work interval. On completion of the eighth interval, take a complete rest – you have earned it.

HIIT/CLASSIC TABATA REGIMEN
Workout 2
Develop: anaerobic threshold, VO2max capacity, fast-twitch fibres and increase EPOC effect.
Workout difficulty: 1

Exercise	Sets	Work Intervals	Rest Intervals	Intensity	Total Time
Boxer Uppercuts	8	20 Sec	10 Sec	Ultra-High	4 Minutes

When using as a standalone workout, include warm-up (five-to-ten minutes), cool-down and stretch (four-to-five minutes). Warm-up time will be specific to your requirements and conditions. Cool-down and stretching time varies and depends on the stretch focus (maintenance or development). Read more on warm-up p.173, cool-down and stretching p.177. Alternatively, filter this workout directly into your existing program (with the assumption that you have already warmed up).

Visual exercise reference
Warm-up exercises   175
Fast and Loose Uppercuts   107

Exercise Guide Note: the Tabata workout consists of 8 x 20-second intervals interspersed with 10-second rest periods. Each interval should be approached with maximum intensity (see RPE chart). Use the rest periods to recover as much as possible before exploding into the next work interval. On completion of the eighth interval, take a complete rest – you have earned it.

HIIT/CLASSIC TABATA REGIMEN

Workout 3

Develop: anaerobic threshold, VO2max capacity, fast-twitch fibres and increase EPOC effect.

Workout difficulty: 1

Exercise	Sets	Work Intervals	Rest Intervals	Intensity	Total Time
Boxer Straight Shots	8	20 Sec	10 Sec	Ultra-High	4 Minutes

When using as a standalone workout, include warm-up (five-to-ten-minutes), cool-down and stretch (four-to-five minutes). Warm-up time will be specific to your requirements and conditions. Cool-down and stretching time varies and depends on the stretch focus (maintenance or development). Read more on warm-up p.173, cool-down and stretching p.177. Alternatively, filter this workout directly into your existing program (with the assumption that you have already warmed up).

Visual exercise reference

Warm-up exercises   175
Fast and Loose Straight Shots   108

Exercise Guide Note: the Tabata workout consists of 8 x 20-second intervals interspersed with 10-second rest periods. Each interval should be approached with maximum intensity (see RPE chart). Use the rest periods to recover as much as possible before exploding into the next work interval. On completion of the eighth interval, take a complete rest – you have earned it.

HIIT/CLASSIC TABATA REGIMEN
Workout 4
Develop: anaerobic threshold, VO2max capacity, fast-twitch fibres and increase EPOC effect.
Workout difficulty: 2

Exercise	Sets	Work Intervals	Rest Intervals	Intensity	Total Time
Side-to-side Squat	8	20 Sec	10 Sec	Ultra-High	4 Minutes

When using as a standalone workout, include warm-up (five-to-ten minutes), cool-down and stretch (four-to-five minutes). Warm-up time will be specific to your requirements and conditions. Cool-down and stretching time varies and depends on the stretch focus (maintenance or development). Read more on warm-up p.173, cool-down and stretching p.177. Alternatively, filter this workout directly into your existing program (with the assumption that you have already warmed up).

Visual exercise reference

Exercise Guide Note: the Tabata workout consists of 8 x 20-second intervals interspersed with 10-second rest periods. Each interval should be approached with maximum intensity (see RPE chart). Use the rest periods to recover as much as possible before exploding into the next work interval. On completion of the eighth interval, take a complete rest – you have earned it.

HIIT/CLASSIC TABATA REGIMEN
Workout 5
Develop: anaerobic threshold, VO2max capacity, fast-twitch fibres and increase EPOC effect.
Workout difficulty: 2

Exercise	Sets	Work Intervals	Rest Intervals	Intensity	Total Time
High Knees	8	20 Sec	10 Sec	Ultra-High	4 Minutes

When using as a standalone workout, include warm-up (five-to-ten minutes), cool-down and stretch (four-to-five minutes). Warm-up time will be specific to your requirements and conditions. Cool-down and stretching time varies and depends on the stretch focus (maintenance or development). Read more on warm-up p.173, cool-down and stretching p.177. Alternatively, filter this workout directly into your existing program (with the assumption that you have already warmed up).

Visual exercise reference
Warm-up exercises   175
High Knees   125

Exercise Guide Note: the Tabata workout consists of 8 x 20-second intervals interspersed with 10-second rest periods. Each interval should be approached with maximum intensity (see RPE chart). Use the rest periods to recover as much as possible before exploding into the next work interval. On completion of the eighth interval, take a complete rest – you have earned it.

HIIT/CLASSIC TABATA REGIMEN
Workout 6
Develop: anaerobic threshold, VO2max capacity, fast-twitch fibres and increase EPOC effect.
Workout difficulty: 3

Exercise	Sets	Work Intervals	Rest Intervals	Intensity	Total Time
Mountain Climber	8	20 Sec	10 Sec	Ultra–High	4 Minutes

When using as a standalone workout, include warm-up (five-to-ten minutes), cool-down and stretch (four-to-five minutes). Warm-up time will be specific to your requirements and conditions. Cool-down and stretching time varies and depends on the stretch focus (maintenance or development). Read more on warm-up p.173, cool-down and stretching p.177. Alternatively, filter this workout directly into your existing program (with the assumption that you have already warmed up).

Visual exercise reference
Warm-up exercises   175
Mountain Climber   126

Exercise Guide Note: the Tabata workout consists of 8 x 20-second intervals interspersed with 10-second rest periods. Each interval should be approached with maximum intensity (see RPE chart). Use the rest periods to recover as much as possible before exploding into the next work interval. On completion of the eighth interval, take a complete rest – you have earned it.

HIIT/CLASSIC TABATA REGIMEN
Workout 7
Develop: anaerobic threshold, VO2max capacity, fast-twitch fibres and increase EPOC effect.
Workout difficulty: 3

Exercise	Sets	Work Intervals	Rest Intervals	Intensity	Total Work-out Time
Burpee	8	20 Sec	10 Sec	Ultra-High	4 Minutes

When using as a standalone workout, include warm-up (five-to-ten minutes), cool-down and stretch (four-to-five minutes). Warm-up time will be specific to your requirements and conditions. Cool-down and stretching time varies and depends on the stretch focus (maintenance or development). Read more on warm-up p.173, cool-down and stretching p.177. Alternatively, filter this workout directly into your existing program (with the assumption that you have already warmed up).

Visual exercise reference
Warm-up exercises   175
Burpee   120

Exercise Guide Note: the Tabata workout consists of 8 x 20-second intervals interspersed with 10-second rest periods. Each interval should be approached with maximum intensity (see RPE chart). Use the rest periods to recover as much as possible before exploding into the next work interval. On completion of the eighth interval, take a complete rest – you have earned it.

HIIT/ALTERNATE TABATA
Workout 8
Develop: anaerobic threshold, VO2max capacity, fast-twitch fibres and increase EPOC effect.
Workout difficulty: 1

Exercise	Sets	Work Intervals	Rest Intervals	Intensity	Total Workout Time
Jumping Jacks	8	20 Sec	10 Sec	High 6–7 RPE	
Boxer Straight Shots	8	20 Sec	10 Sec	High 6–7 RPE	8 Minutes

When using as a standalone workout, include warm-up (five-to-ten minutes), cool-down and stretch (four-to-five minutes). Warm-up time will be specific to your requirements and conditions. Cool-down and stretching time varies and depends on the stretch focus (maintenance or development). Read more on warm-up p.173, cool-

down and stretching p.177. Alternatively, filter this workout directly into your existing program (with the assumption that you have already warmed up).

Visual exercise reference

Warm-up exercises	175
Jumping Jack	110
Fast and Loose Straight Shots	108

Exercise Guide Note: this Alternate Tabata workout consists of 16 x 20-second intervals interspersed with 10-second rest periods. Alternate between exercises: Jumping Jack, Fast and Loose Straight Shots, Jumping Jack and so on. Continue until 16 work intervals are complete. Maintain a consistent high level of intensity – approximately 6-7 on the RPE chart (maximal intensity with this volume of work is unrealistic). If you can sustain a higher level throughout, do so.

HIIT/ALTERNATE TABATA
Workout 9
Develop: anaerobic threshold, VO2max capacity, fast-twitch fibres and increase EPOC effect.
Workout difficulty: 2

Exercise	Sets	Work Intervals	Rest Intervals	Intensity	Total Workout time
Side-to-side squats	8	20 Sec	10 Sec	High 6–7 RPE	

Boxer Uppercuts	8	20 Sec	10 Sec	High 6-7 RPE	
					8 Minutes

When using as a standalone workout, include warm-up (five to-ten minutes), cool-down and stretch (four-to-five minutes). Warm-up time will be specific to your requirements and conditions. Cool-down and stretching time varies and depends on the stretch focus (maintenance or development). Read more on warm-up p.173, cool-down and stretching p.177. Alternatively, filter this workout directly into your existing program (with the assumption that you have already warmed up).

Visual exercise reference

Warm-up exercises	175
Side-to-Side Squats	114
Fast and Loose Uppercuts	107

Exercise Guide Note: this Alternate Tabata workout consists of 16 x 20-second intervals interspersed with 10-second rest periods. Alternate between exercises: Side-to-side Squats, Fast and Loose Uppercuts and so on. Continue until 16 work intervals are complete. Maintain a consistent high level of intensity – approximately 6–7 on the RPE Chart (maximal intensity with this volume of work is unrealistic). If you can sustain a higher level throughout, do so.

HIIT/ALTERNATE TABATA

Workout 10

Develop: anaerobic threshold, VO2max capacity, fast-twitch fibres and increase EPOC effect.

Workout difficulty: 3

Exercise	Sets	Work Intervals	Rest Intervals	Intensity	Total Workout time
Burpee	8	20 Sec	10 Sec	High 6–7 RPE	
Jumping Jack	8	20 Sec	10 Sec	High 6–7 RPE	8 minutes

When using as a standalone workout, include warm-up (five-to-ten minutes), cool-down and stretch (four-to-five minutes). Warm-up time will be specific to your requirements and conditions. Cool-down and stretching time varies and depends on the stretch focus (maintenance or development). Read more on warm-up p.173, cool-down and stretching p.177. Alternatively, filter this workout directly into your existing program (with the assumption that you have already warmed up).

Visual exercise reference

Warm-up exercises   175
Burpee   120
Jumping Jack   110

Exercise Guide Note: this Alternate Tabata workout consists of 16 x 20-second intervals interspersed with 10-second rest periods. Alternate between exercises: Burpee, Jumping Jack, Burpee and so on. Continue until 16 work intervals are complete. Maintain a consistent high level of intensity – approximately 6–7 on the RPE Chart (maximal intensity with this volume of work is unrealistic). If you can sustain a higher level throughout, do so.

HIIT/ALTERNATE TABATA

Workout 11

Develop: anaerobic threshold, VO2max capacity, fast-twitch fibres and increase EPOC effect.

Workout difficulty: 3

Exercise	Sets	Work Intervals	Rest Intervals	Intensity	Total Workout time
Prisoner Squat	8	20 Sec	10 Sec	High 6–7 RPE	
Press–Up	8	20 Sec	10 Sec	High 6–7 RPE	8 minutes

When using as a standalone workout, include warm-up (five-to-ten minutes), cool-down and stretch (four-to-five minutes). Warm-up time will be specific to your requirements and conditions. Cool-down and stretching time varies and depends on the stretch focus (maintenance or development). Read more on warm-up p.173, cool-

down and stretching p.177. Alternatively, filter this workout directly into your existing program (with the assumption that you have already warmed up).

Visual exercise reference

Warm-up exercises	175
Prisoner Squat	69
Press-Up	48

Exercise Guide Note: this Alternate Tabata workout consists of 16 x 20-second intervals interspersed with 10-second rest periods. Alternate between exercises: Prisoner Squat, Press-up, Prisoner Squat and so on. Continue until 16 work intervals are complete. Maintain a consistent high level of intensity – approximately 6–7 on the RPE Chart (maximal intensity with this volume of work is unrealistic). If you can sustain a higher level throughout, do so.

HIIT/MULTI-TABATA
Workout 12
Develop: anaerobic threshold, VO2max capacity, fast-twitch fibres and increase EPOC effect
Workout difficulty: 4

Exercise	Sets	Work	Rest	Intensity	Total Workout time
Boxer Straight Shots	8	20 Sec	10 Sec	High 6–7 RPE	

Wide Squats	8	20 Sec	10 Sec	High 6–7 RPE	
Boxer Uppercuts	8	20 Sec	10 Sec	High 6–7 RPE	
Dolphin Press-Up	8	20 Sec	10 Sec	High 6–7 RPE	
					16 Minutes

When using as a standalone workout, include warm-up (five-to-ten minutes), cool-down and stretch (four-to-five minutes). Warm-up time will be specific to your requirements and conditions. Cool-down and stretching time varies and depends on the stretch focus (maintenance or development). Read more on warm-up p.173, cool-down and stretching p.177. Alternatively, filter this workout directly into your existing program (with the assumption that you have already warmed up).

Visual exercise reference

Warm-up exercises	175
Fast and Loose Straight Shots	108
Wide Squat	68
Fast and Loose Uppercuts	107
Dolphin Press-Up	50

Exercise Guide Note: this Multi-Tabata workout consists of 32 x 20-second intervals interspersed with 10-second rest periods. Complete eight sets of one exercise before moving onto the next exercise – example: finish all Boxer Straight Shots before moving onto Wide Squats, until all 32 work intervals are completed. Maintain a consistent high level of intensity – approximately 6–7 on the RPE chart (maximal intensity with this volume of work is unrealistic). If you can sustain a higher level throughout, do so.

HIIT/MULTI-TABATA
Workout 13
Develop: anaerobic threshold, VO2max capacity, fast-twitch fibres and increase EPOC effect.
Workout difficulty: 4

Exercise	Sets	Work Intervals	Rest Intervals	Intensity	Total Workout Time
Jumping Jack	8	20 Sec	10 Sec	High 6–7 RPE	
Prisoner Squat	8	20 Sec	10 Sec	High 6–7 RPE	
Jumping Jack	8	20 Sec	10 Sec	High 6–7 RPE	
Mountain Climber	8	20 Sec	10 Sec	High 6–7 RPE	16 Minutes

When using as a standalone workout, include warm-up (five-to-ten minutes), cool-down and stretch (four-to-five minutes). Warm-up time will be specific to your requirements and conditions. Cool-down and stretching time varies and depends on the stretch focus (maintenance or development). Read more on warm-up p.173, cool-

down and stretching p.177. Alternatively, filter this workout directly into your existing program (with the assumption that you have already warmed up).

Visual exercise reference

Exercise Guide Note: this Multi-Tabata workout consists of 32 x 20-second intervals interspersed with 10-second rest periods. Complete eight sets of one exercise before moving onto the next exercise – example: finish all Jumping Jacks before moving onto Prisoner Squats, until all 32 work intervals are completed. Maintain a consistent high level of intensity – approximately 6–7 on the RPE chart (maximal intensity with this volume of work is unrealistic). If you can sustain a higher level throughout, do so.

HIIT/MULTI-TABATA
Workout 14
Develop: anaerobic threshold, VO2max capacity, fast-twitch fibres and increase EPOC effect.
Exercise difficulty: 4

WORKOUTS AND PROGRAMS

Exercise	Sets	Work Intervals	Rest Intervals	Intensity	Total Workout time
Burpee with Press-up	8	20 Sec	10 Sec	High 6–7 RPE	
Boxer Uppercuts	8	20 Sec	10 Sec	High 6–7 RPE	
Mountain Climber	8	20 Sec	10 Sec	High 6–7 RPE	
Jumping Jack	8	20 Sec	10 Sec	High 6–7 RPE	
					16 Minutes

When using as a standalone workout, include warm-up (five-to-ten minutes), cool-down and stretch (four-to-five minutes). Warm-up time will be specific to your requirements and conditions. Cool-down and stretching time varies and depends on the stretch focus (maintenance or development). Read more on warm-up p.173, cool-down and stretching p.177. Alternatively, filter this workout directly into your existing program (with the assumption that you have already warmed up).

Visual exercise reference

Exercise Guide Note: this Multi-Tabata workout consists of 32 x 20-second intervals interspersed with 10-second rest periods. Complete eight sets of one exercise before moving onto the next exercise – example: finish all Burpees with Press-ups before moving onto Fast and Loose Uppercuts, until all 32 work intervals are completed. Maintain a consistent high level of intensity – approximately 6–7 on the RPE chart (maximal intensity with this volume of work is unrealistic). If you can sustain a higher level throughout, do so.

GPP WORKOUTS

Read more on GPP Workouts on p.23

Guide

The GPP HIIT workouts are expressed with different work-to-rest ratios, adding variety to training stimulus. The initial workouts present a 3:1 ratio of three minutes' work to one minute's rest; the following workouts are a 2:1 (40w/20r and 30w/15r, respectively), with the final Warrior Challenge combining reps with time. In all cases, the aim is to train at a high intensity with the focus on consistency, maintaining output.

Frequency: one to two times per week (dependent on other HIIT workouts in a given week).

Equipment

A stopwatch is required as these are timed workouts. There are several free stopwatch Apps available. I recommend a (currently) free timer called 'Interval Timer' for the iPhone, designed by Deltaworks (there are lots to choose from). Alternatively, for Android, download the (currently) free 'Stopwatch and Timer' App, designed by sportstracklive.com.

Approach

GPP workouts should be approached at a high but sub-maximal intensity. Strive to maintain a level of approximately 6–7 on the RPE chart.

Use the Rate of Perceived Exertion Chart below to measure your intensity level:

Borg CR10 Scale

0	No exertion at all	
0.5	Extremely light	
1	Very light	
2	Fairly light	
3	Moderate	
4	Somewhat hard	
5	Hard	
6		
7	Very hard	GPP Zone
8		
9		
10	Extremely hard	
*	Maximal	

(Intensity / Effort)

Workout difficulty level

Each workout has a 'workout difficulty' number – the higher the number the more challenging the workout.

Progressions

Strive to increase intensity output for longer periods of time. Add reps, sets and cycles where necessary. Continue to push your upper levels, aiming to work harder for longer.

Caution: these programs are not suitable for beginners – a solid fitness background is required before taking part. If you are untrained, sedentary, have underlying health problems or biomechanical issues, it is inadvisable to participate at this level of activity, as there is an increased risk of injury. If in doubt, seek medical advice before attempting any of the workouts.

HIIT/GPP RATIO 3:1 (180W/60R)

Workout 1

Develop: anaerobic threshold, VO2max capacity, muscle endurance and increase EPOC effect.

Workout difficulty: 2

Exercise	Continuous Work Intervals	Intensity RPE Chart	Rest Between Circuits	Circuits	Total Workout (Approximate)
Boxer Uppercuts	30 Sec	High 6-7	60 Sec	3-5	
Jumping Jack	30 Sec	High 6-7			
Squat	30 Sec	High 6-7			
Jumping Jack	30 Sec	High 6-7			
Boxer Straight Shots	30 Sec	High 6-7			
Standard Press-Up	30 Sec	High 6-7			
1 Circuit					
					11-19 minutes

When using as a standalone workout, include warm-up (five-to-ten minutes), cool-down and stretch (four-to-five minutes). Warm-up time will be specific to your requirements and conditions. Cool-down and stretching time varies and depends on the stretch focus (maintenance or development). Read more on warm-up p.173, cool-down and stretching p.177. Alternatively, filter this workout directly into your existing program (with the assumption that you have already warmed up).

Visual exercise reference

Warm-up exercises	175
Fast and Loose Uppercuts	107
Jumping Jack	110
Standard Squat	66
Fast and Loose Straight Shots	108
Standard Press-up	48

Exercise Guide Note: this high-intensity GPP 3:1 ratio (three minutes' work, one minute's rest) circuit should be approached at intensity 6–7 on the RPE chart. Perform all 30-second work intervals without stopping. When all six intervals are complete, this constitutes one circuit. Perform three to five circuits, resting for 60 seconds between each one.

HIIT/GPP RATIO 3:1 (180W/60R)
Workout 2
Develop: anaerobic threshold, VO2max capacity, muscle endurance and increase EPOC effect.
Workout difficulty: 2

Exercise	Continuous Work Intervals	Intensity RPE Chart	Rest Between Circuits	Circuits	Total Workout (Approximate)
Jumping Jack	30 Sec	High 6–7	60 Sec	3–5	
Alternate Lunge	30 Sec	High 6–7			
Mountain Climber	30 Sec	High 6–7			
Jumping Jack	30 Sec	High 6–7			
Wide Squat	30 Sec	High 6–7			
Mountain Climber	30 Sec	High 6–7			
1 Circuit					
					11–19 Minutes

When using as a standalone workout, include warm-up (five-to-ten minutes), cool-down and stretch (four-to-five minutes). Warm-up time will be specific to your requirements and conditions. Cool-down and stretching time varies and depends on the stretch focus (maintenance or development). Read more on warm-up p.173, cool-down and stretching p.177. Alternatively, filter this workout directly into your existing program (with the assumption that you have already warmed up).

Visual exercise reference

Warm-up exercises	175
Jumping Jack	110
Alternate Lunge	73
Mountain Climber	126
Wide Squat	68

Exercise Guide Note: this high-intensity GPP 3:1 ratio (three minutes' work, one minute's rest) circuit should be approached at intensity 6–7 on the RPE chart. Perform all 30-second work intervals without stopping. When all six intervals are complete, this constitutes one circuit. Perform three to five circuits, resting for 60 seconds between each one.

HIIT/GPP RATIO 3:1 (180W/60R)

Workout 3

Develop: anaerobic threshold, VO2max capacity, muscle endurance and increase EPOC effect.

Workout difficulty: 3

Exercise	Continuous Work Intervals	Intensity RPE Chart	Rest Between Circuits	Circuits	Total Workout (Approximate)
Burpee with Press-up	30 Sec	High 6-7	60 Sec	3-5	
Jumping Jack	30 Sec	High 6-7			
Side-to-Side Squat	30 Sec	High 6-7			
Burpee with Press-up	30 Sec	High 6-7			
Jumping Jack	30 Sec	High 6-7			
Pike Shoulder Press	30 Sec	High 6-7			
1 Circuit					
					11-19 Minutes

When using as a standalone workout, include warm-up (five-to-ten minutes), cool-down and stretch (four-to-five minutes). Warm-up time will be specific to your requirements and conditions. Cool-down and stretching time varies and depends on the stretch focus (maintenance or development). Read more on warm-up p.173, cool-down and stretching p.177. Alternatively, filter this workout directly into your existing program (with the assumption that you have already warmed up).

Visual exercise reference

Warm-up exercises	175
Burpee with Press-Up	122
Jumping Jack	110
Side-to-Side Squat	114
Pike Shoulder Press-Up	57

Exercise Guide Note: this high-intensity GPP 3:1 ratio (three minutes' work, one minute's rest) circuit should be approached at intensity 6–7 on the RPE chart. Perform all 30-second work intervals without stopping. When all six intervals are complete, this constitutes one circuit. Perform three to five circuits, resting for 60 seconds between each one.

HIIT/GPP RATIO 3:1 (180W/60R)
Workout 4
Develop: anaerobic threshold, VO2max capacity, muscle endurance and increase EPOC effect.
Workout difficulty: 3

Exercise	Continuous Work Intervals	Intensity RPE Chart	Rest Between Circuits	Circuits	Total Workout (Approximate)
Squat Jump	30 Sec	High 6–7	60 Sec	3–5	
Boxer Uppercuts	30 Sec	High 6–7			
Spider-Man Press-Up	30 Sec	High 6–7			
Squat Jump	30 Sec	High 6–7			
Boxer Uppercuts	30 Sec	High 6–7			
Dolphin Press-Up	30 Sec	High 6–7			
1 Circuit					
					11–19 minutes

When using as a standalone workout, include warm-up (five-to-ten minutes), cool-down and stretch (four-to-five minutes). Warm-up time will be specific to your requirements and conditions. Cool-down and stretching time varies and depends on the stretch focus (maintenance or development). Read more on warm-up p.173, cool-

down and stretching p.177. Alternatively, filter this workout directly into your existing program (with the assumption that you have already warmed up).

Visual exercise reference

Warm-up exercises	175
Squat Jump	113
Fast and Loose Uppercuts	107
Spider-Man Press-Up	53
Dolphin Press-Up	50

Exercise Guide Note: This high-intensity GPP 3:1 ratio (three minutes' work, one minute's rest) circuit should be approached at intensity 6–7 on the RPE chart. Perform all 30-second work intervals without stopping. When all six intervals are complete, this constitutes one circuit. Perform three to five circuits, resting for 60 seconds between each one.

HIIT/GPP RATIO 3:1 (180W/60R)
Workout 5
Develop: anaerobic threshold, VO2max capacity, muscle endurance and increase EPOC effect.
Workout difficulty: 4

Exercise	Continuous Work Intervals	Intensity RPE Chart	Rest Between Circuits	Circuits	Total Workout (Approximate)
Burpee, Press-Up and Tuck Jump	30 Sec	High 6–7	60 Sec	3–5	

Jumping Jack	30 Sec	High 6–7			
Boxing Shuffle	30 Sec	High 6–7			
Burpee, Press-Up and Tuck Jump	30 Sec	High 6–7			
Jumping Jack	30 Sec	High 6–7			
Standard Press-Up	30 Sec	High 6–7			
1 Circuit					
				11–19 minutes	

When using as a standalone workout, include warm-up (five-to-ten minutes), cool-down and stretch (four-to-five minutes). Warm-up time will be specific to your requirements and conditions. Cool-down and stretching time varies and depends on the stretch focus (maintenance or development). Read more on warm-up P.173, cool-down and stretching P.177. Alternatively, filter this workout directly into your existing program (with the assumption that you have already warmed up).

Visual exercise reference

Exercise Guide Note: this high-intensity GPP 3:1 ratio (three minutes' work, one minute's rest) circuit should be approached at intensity 6–7 on the RPE chart. Perform all 30-second work intervals without stopping. When all six intervals are complete, this constitutes one circuit. Perform three to five circuits, resting for 60 seconds between each one.

HIIT/GPP RATIO 2:1 (40W/20R)

Workout 6

Develop: anaerobic threshold, VO2max capacity, muscle endurance and increase EPOC effect.

Workout difficulty: 3

Exercise	High-Intensity Work Interval	Low-Intensity Work Interval	Cycles	Total Workout Time (Approximate)
Mountain Climber	40 Sec RPE 6–7		4–10	
Boxing Shuffle		20 Sec RPE 2–3		

1 Cycle		
		4–10 minutes

When using as a standalone workout, include warm-up (five-to-ten minutes), cool-down and stretch (four-to-five minutes). Warm-up time will be specific to your requirements and conditions. Cool-down and stretching time varies and depends on the stretch focus (maintenance or development). Read more on warm-up p.173, cool-down and stretching p.177. Alternatively, filter this workout directly into your existing program (with the assumption that you have already warmed up).

Visual exercise reference
Warm-up exercises   175
Mountain Climber   126
Boxing Shuffle   109

Exercise Guide Note:
This high-intensity GPP 2:1 ratio involves a 40-second high-intensity interval at 6–7 on the RPE chart, followed by a 20-second low-intensity interval at 2–3 on the RPE chart. This constitutes one cycle performed between four-to-ten cycles without stopping. Use the low-intensity interval as 'active rest'.

HIIT/GPP RATIO 2:1 (40W/20R)
Workout 7
Develop: anaerobic threshold, VO2max capacity, muscle endurance and increase EPOC effect.
Workout difficulty: 3

Exercise	High-Intensity Work Interval	Low-Intensity Work Interval	Cycles	Total Workout Time (Approximate)
Burpee	40 Sec RPE 6-7		4-10	
Boxer Uppercuts		20 Sec RPE 2-3		
1 Cycle				
				4-10 minutes

When using as a standalone workout, include warm-up (five-to-ten minutes), cool-down and stretch (four-to-five minutes). Warm-up time will be specific to your requirements and conditions. Cool-down and stretching time varies and depends on the stretch focus (maintenance or development). Read more on warm-up p.173, cool-down and stretching p.177. Alternatively, filter this workout directly into your existing program (with the assumption that you have already warmed up).

Visual exercise reference

This high-intensity GPP 2:1 ratio involves a 40-second high-intensity interval at 6–7 on the RPE chart, followed by a 20-second low-intensity interval at 2–3 on the RPE chart. This constitutes one cycle performed between four-to-ten cycles without stopping. Use the low-intensity interval as 'active rest'.

HIIT/GPP RATIO 2:1 (40W/20R)

Workout 8

Develop: anaerobic threshold, VO2max capacity, muscle endurance and increase EPOC effect.

Workout difficulty: 3

Exercise	High–Intensity Work Interval	Low–Intensity Work Interval	Cycles	Total Workout Time (Approximate)
Burpee with Press–Up	40 Sec RPE 6–7		4–10	
Boxer Straight Shots		20 Sec RPE 2–3		
1 Cycle				
				4–10 Minutes

When using as a standalone workout, include warm-up (five-to-ten minutes), cool-down and stretch (four-to-five minutes). Warm-up time will be specific to your requirements and conditions. Cool-down and stretching time varies and depends on the stretch focus (maintenance or development). Read more on warm-up p.173, cool-down and stretching p.177. Alternatively, filter this workout directly into your existing program (with the assumption that you have already warmed up).

Visual exercise reference

Warm-up exercises   175

Burpee with Press-Up   122

Fast and Loose Straight Shots   108

This high-intensity GPP 2:1 ratio involves a 40-second high-intensity interval at 6–7 on the RPE chart, followed by a 20-second low-intensity interval at 2–3 on the RPE chart. This constitutes one cycle performed between four-to-ten cycles without stopping. Use the low-intensity interval as 'active rest'.

HIIT/GPP RATIO 2:1 (30W/15R)
Workout 9
Develop: anaerobic threshold, VO2max capacity, muscle endurance and increase EPOC effect.
Workout difficulty: 3

Exercise	High-Intensity Work Interval	Low-Intensity Work Interval	Cycles	Total Workout Time (Approximate)
High Knees	30 Sec RPE 7–8		4–10	

Boxer Straight Shots		15 Sec RPE 2–3		
1 Cycle				
				4–10 minutes

When using as a standalone workout, include warm-up (five to ten 10 minutes), cool-down and stretch (four-to-five minutes). Warm-up time will be specific to your requirements and conditions. Cool-down and stretching time varies and depends on the stretch focus (maintenance or development). Read more on warm-up p.173, cool-down and stretching p.177. Alternatively, filter this workout directly into your existing program (with the assumption that you have already warmed up).

Visual exercise reference

Warm-up exercises	175
High Knees	125
Fast and Loose Straight Shots	108

Exercise Guide Note: this high-intensity GPP 2:1 ratio involves a 30-second high-intensity interval at 7–8 on the RPE chart, followed by a 15-second low-intensity interval at 2–3 on the RPE Chart. This constitutes one cycle performed between four-to-ten cycles without stopping. Use the low-intensity interval as 'active rest'.

HIIT/GPP RATIO 2:1 (30W/15R)

Workout 10

Develop: anaerobic threshold, VO2max capacity, muscle endurance and increase EPOC effect.

Workout difficulty: 4

Exercise	High-Intensity Work Interval	Low-Intensity Work Interval	Cycles	Total Workout Time (Approximate)
Burpee, Press-Up and Tuck Jump	30 Sec RPE 7–8		4–10	
Boxer Shuffle		15 Sec RPE 2–3		
1 Cycle				
				4–10 minutes

When using as a standalone workout, include warm-up (five-to-ten-minutes), cool-down and stretch (four-to-five minutes). Warm-up time will be specific to your requirements and conditions. Cool-down and stretching time varies and depends on the stretch focus (maintenance or development). Read more on warm-up p.173, cool-down and stretching p.177. Alternatively, filter this workout directly into your existing program (with the assumption that you have already warmed up).

Visual exercise reference

Exercise Guide Note: this high-intensity GPP 2:1 ratio involves a 30-second high-intensity interval at 7–8 on the RPE chart, followed by a 15-second low-intensity interval at 2–3 on the RPE Chart. This constitutes one cycle performed between four-to-ten cycles without stopping. Use the low-intensity interval as 'active rest'.

HIIT/GPP WARRIOR INTERVALS

Workout 11

Develop: anaerobic threshold, VO2max capacity, muscle endurance and increase EPOC effect.

Workout difficulty: 4

Exercise	Repetitions /Time	Tempo/ Intensity	Rest Between Cycles	Cycles	Total Workout Time (Approximate)
Spider-Man Press-Up	18–20	2	60 Sec	1–3	
Jumping Jack	60 Sec	High 6–7 RPE			
Wide Squat	15–20	3			

Mountain Climber	60 Sec	High 6–7 RPE			
Pike Shoulder Press-Up	15–20	2			
Jumping Jack	60 Sec	High 6–7 RPE			
RDL	10 Per Leg	3			
Mountain Climber	60 Sec	High 6–7			
1 Cycle					
					6–20 Minutes

When using as a standalone workout, include warm-up (five-to-ten minutes), cool-down and stretch (four-to-five minutes). Warm-up time will be specific to your requirements and conditions. Cool-down and stretching time varies and depends on the stretch focus (maintenance or development). Read more on warm-up p.173, cool-down and stretching p.177. Alternatively, filter this workout directly into your existing program (with the assumption that you have already warmed up).

Visual exercise reference
Warm-up exercises   175

Pike Shoulder Press-Up	57
Spider-Man Press-Up	53
Single-Leg RDL	78
Jumping Jack	110
Wide Squat	68
Mountain Climber	126

Exercise Guide Note: GPP Warrior Intervals consist of reps and tempo count followed by time intervals at 6–7 RPE. Each exercise must be executed continuously without stopping. Once all exercises are complete, this will constitute one cycle. Perform one to three cycles. Rest for 60 seconds between cycles.

Note: The tempo count represents the number you count concentrically (when the muscle shortens) and the number you count eccentrically (when the muscle lengthens). Therefore, a 'three' is more intense than a 'two', as the muscles are under tension for longer; a 'four' would constitute even more intensity. Set your level so that 10–12 reps becomes challenging. Rest between sets, as prescribed, or adjust according to your needs.

HIIT/GPP WARRIOR INTERVALS
Workout 12
Develop: anaerobic threshold, VO2max capacity, muscle endurance and increase EPOC effect.
Workout difficulty: 4

WORKOUTS AND PROGRAMS

Exercise	Repetitions /Time	Tempo/ Intensity	Rest Between Cycles	Cycles	Total Workout Time (Approximate)
Knuckle Press-Up	18–20	2	60 Sec	1–3	
Boxer Shuffle	60 Sec	High 6–7 RPE			
Prisoner Squat	15–20	3			
Burpee Shuffle	60 Sec	High 6–7 RPE			
Decline Press-Up	15–20	2			
Boxer Shuffle	60 Sec	High 6–7 RPE			
Bulgarian Squat	10 Per Leg	3			
Burpee	60 Sec	High 6–7			
1 Cycle					
					6–20 minutes

When using as a standalone workout, include warm-up (five-to-ten minutes), cool-down and stretch (four-to-five minutes). Warm-up time will be specific to your requirements and conditions. Cool-down and stretching time varies and depends on the stretch focus (maintenance or development). Read more on warm-up p.173, cool-down and stretching p.177. Alternatively, filter this workout directly into your existing program (with the assumption that you have already warmed up).

Visual exercise reference

Warm-up exercises	175
Decline Press-Up	57
Knuckle Press-Up	55
Bulgarian Squat	70
Boxing Shuffle	109
Prisoner Squat	69
Burpee	120

Exercise Guide Note: GPP Warrior Intervals consist of reps and tempo count followed by time intervals at 6–7 RPE. Each exercise must be executed continuously without stopping. Once all exercises are complete, this will constitute one cycle. Perform one to three cycles. Rest for sixty 60 seconds between cycles.

Note: The tempo count represents the number you count concentrically (when the muscle shortens) and the number you count eccentrically (when the muscle lengthens). Therefore, a 'three' is more intense than a 'two', as the muscles are under tension for longer; a 'four' would constitute even more intensity. Set your level so that 10–12 reps becomes challenging. Rest between sets, as prescribed, or adjust according to your needs.

RESISTANCE WORKOUTS

Read more on Resistance Workouts on page 24

Guide

This section contains resistance rapid-workouts aimed at hypertrophy (muscle growth) and muscular endurance. There is an initial workout for those with less upper-body strength that can be modified to suit the individual. The other workouts allow for those with existing muscular strength (from regular to high) and have emphasis on either growth or endurance and, for some participants, maximal strength (depending on their current level). There are upper-body and lower-body workouts, as well as combination workouts.

Frequency: two-to-three times per week (dependent on other resistance workouts in a given week). Forty-eight hours rest between body parts. (No equipment is required for these workouts.)

Approach

Execute all exercises with proper form, as described. Focus on the main-target muscle, as listed in the exercise description. In doing so, you sustain the integrity of the exercise, keeping the effort concentrated on the intended target (there are, of course, synergists assisting movement but our focus here is on the prime mover).

Workout difficulty level

This number appears on each workout and refers to the overall level of difficulty for a given workout, as prescribed. However, the level of intensity can be increased or decreased depending on your current level of ability and to match the specific training target. Adjustment to tempo (speed) when executing an exercise will have a direct impact on how difficult or easy an exercise becomes.

Progressions

The workouts can be made more intense by altering the tempo of execution and/or exchanging the prescribed exercise for a more challenging variety – for example, pike press-up: progress to a decline pike press-up. In addition, one can change the *format* of the workout itself; where a workout is prescribed in sets with rests (i.e. three to four sets with 30-to-60 seconds' rest), you could instead attempt all the exercises consecutively, performing one set per exercise without rest. On completion of the circuit, take a rest (60-to-90 seconds) before completing further circuits. Be imaginative and continue to exchange exercises and experiment with tempo – remember that our body responds to progressions, the changing stimuli and resultant adaptations.

For those finding specific exercises or workouts too much of a challenge, remember that an exercise can be modified into an easier version by altering the ROM (range of motion) and making the movement shorter. For example, a partial press-up would involve descending to mid-range only and pressing back up. Alternatively, selecting an easier exercise (extended-kneeling press-up) is another option. Workouts can be made easier by reducing reps and sets and increasing rest time. The most important factor is that we aim to keep in sync with the exercise target of any given workout, so that any modifications, changes or alterations that need to be made to fulfil that goal in terms of exercises, tempo and rest are made.

Caution: these programs are not suitable for beginners – a solid fitness background is required before taking part. If you are untrained, sedentary, have underlying health problems or biomechanical issues, it is inadvisable to participate at this level of activity, as there is an increased risk of injury. If in doubt, seek medical advice before attempting any of the workouts.

RESISTANCE STRAIGHT-SETS WORKOUT (ISOTONIC)

Workout 1: Upper Body.

Develop: hypertrophy (muscular growth).

Workout difficulty: 1 (start here if upper-body strength is low).

Exercise	Reps	Sets	Rest (Between Sets)	Tempo (Count)	Total Workout Time (Approximate)
Extended-Kneeling Press-Up	10–12	3–4	45–60 Sec	3	
Negative Press-Up	10–12	3–4	45–60 Sec	3	
Elevated Dip	10–12	3–4	45–60 Sec	3	
					10–15 Minutes

When using as a standalone workout, include warm-up (five-to-ten-minutes), cool-down and stretch (four-to-five minutes). Warm-up time will be specific to your requirements and conditions. Cool-down and stretching time varies and depends on the stretch focus (maintenance or development). Read more on warm-up 173, cool-

down and stretching p.177. Alternatively, filter this workout directly into your existing program (with the assumption that you have already warmed up).

Visual exercise reference

Exercise Guide Note: this resistance workout is targeting a hypertrophy range of 10–12 repetitions, representing varying degrees of difficulty, depending on an individual's current strength level. To ensure you remain within the exercise-repetition target (hypertrophy), adjust your *tempo* accordingly – slowing the movement down will increase the level of intensity. In this instance, tempo has been set at 'three'. This translates to a three count during the concentric phase and the eccentric phase (when the muscles shorten and lengthen under tension). Tempo three may represent the ideal challenge for you; if not, adjust tempo to a four count. Similarly, if too difficult, reduce tempo to two. The rest between sets is displayed as 45–60 seconds (*extend* or *shorten* rest periods specific to your requirements but ensure you take enough rest to replenish the short energy supply). Increase the repetitions to enter *muscular endurance* on the strength continuum.

RESISTANCE STRAIGHT-SETS WORKOUT (ISOTONIC)
Workout 2: Upper Body.
Develop: hypertrophy (muscular growth).
Workout difficulty: 2

Exercise	Reps	Sets	Rest (Between Sets)	Tempo (Count)	Total Workout Time (Approximate)
Standard Press-Up	10–12	3–4	45–60 Sec	3	
Decline Press-Up	10–12	3–4	45–60 Sec	3	
Pike Press-Up	10–12	3–4	45–60 Sec	3	
Double Elevated Dip	10–12	3–4	45–60 Sec	3	12–16 Minutes

When using as a standalone workout, include warm-up (five-to-ten minutes), cool-down and stretch (four-to-five minutes). Warm-up time will be specific to your requirements and conditions. Cool-down and stretching time varies and depends on the stretch focus (maintenance or development). Read more on warm-up p.173, cool-down and stretching p.177. Alternatively, filter this workout directly into your existing program (with the assumption that you have already warmed up).

Visual exercise reference

Exercise Guide Note: this resistance workout is targeting a hypertrophy range of 10–12 repetitions, representing varying degrees of difficulty, depending on an individual's current strength level. To ensure you remain within the exercise-repetition target (hypertrophy), adjust your tempo accordingly – slowing the movement down will increase the level of intensity. In this instance, *tempo* has been set at 'three'.

This translates to a three count during the concentric phase and the eccentric phase (when the muscles shorten and lengthen under tension). Tempo three may represent the ideal challenge for you; if not, adjust tempo to a four count. Similarly, if too difficult, reduce tempo to two. The rest between sets is displayed as 45–60 seconds (*extend* or *shorten* rest periods specific to your requirements but ensure you take enough rest to replenish the short energy supply). Add or reduce sets to suit requirements.

RESISTANCE STRAIGHT-SETS WORKOUT (ISOTONIC)
Workout 3: Upper Body.
Develop: muscular endurance.
Workout difficulty: 2

Exercise	Reps	Sets	Rest (Between Sets)	Tempo (Count)	Total Workout Time (Approximate)
Standard Press-Up	15–20	3–5	30–45 Sec	2	
Decline Press-Up	15–20	3–5	30–45 Sec	2	
Pike Press-Up	15–20	3–5	30–45 Sec	2	
Double Elevated Dip	15–20	3–5	30–45 Sec	2	
					12–20 minutes

When using as a standalone workout, include warm-up (five-to-ten-minutes), cool-down and stretch (four-to-five minutes). Warm-up time will be specific to your requirements and conditions. Cool-down and stretching time varies and depends on the stretch focus (maintenance or development). Read more on warm-up p.173, cool-down and stretching p.177. Alternatively, filter this workout directly into your existing program (with the assumption that you have already warmed up).

Visual exercise reference

Standard Press-Up	48
Double Elevated Dip	64
Decline Press-Up	57

This resistance workout is targeting a muscular endurance range of 15–20 repetitions, representing varying degrees of difficulty depending on an individual's current strength level. To ensure you remain within the exercise repetition target (muscle endurance), adjust your tempo accordingly – slowing the movement down will increase the level of intensity. In this instance, *tempo* has been set at 'two'. This translates as a two count during the concentric phase and the eccentric phase (when the muscles shorten and lengthen under tension).

Tempo two may represent the ideal challenge for you; if not, adjust tempo to a three count to increase intensity. If tempo two is too difficult, *modify the exercise* and replace with an easier alternative (for example, extended-kneeling press-up instead of standard press-up) or shorten the ROM (range of motion). The rest between sets is displayed as 30–45 seconds (*extend* or *shorten* rest periods specific to your requirements but ensure you take enough rest to replenish the short energy supply). Add or reduce sets to suit requirements.

RESISTANCE STRAIGHT-SETS WORKOUT (ISOTONIC)
Workout 4: Upper-Body Fighter's Workout.
Develop: upper-body muscular strength and endurance; strengthen bones of the hands and wrists.
Workout difficulty: 3

Exercise	Reps	Sets	Rest (Between Sets)	Tempo (Count)	Total Workout Time (Approximate)
Knuckle Press-Up	10–12	3–4	45–60 Sec	3	
Spider-Man Press-Up	10–12 Alternate	3–4	45–60 Sec	3	
Decline Pike Press-up	10–12	3–4	45–60 Sec	3	
Double Elevated Dip	10–12	3–4	45–60 Sec	3	
				12–20 Minutes	

When using as a standalone workout, include warm-up (five-to-ten-minutes), cool-down and stretch (four-to-five minutes). Warm-up time will be specific to your requirements and conditions. Cool-down and stretching time varies and depends on the stretch focus (maintenance or development). Read more on warm-up p.173, cool-down and stretching p.177. Alternatively, filter this workout directly into your existing program (with the assumption that you have already warmed up).

Visual exercise reference

Exercise Guide Note: the fighter's resistance workout includes exercises to improve hand, forearm and shoulder strength. Ten-to-twelve reps will represent varying degrees of difficulty, depending on an individual's current strength level. To ensure you remain within the exercise-rep target, adjust your tempo accordingly – slowing the movement down will increase the level of intensity. In this instance, *tempo* has been set at 'three'. This translates to a three count during the concentric phase and the eccentric phase (when the muscles shorten and lengthen under tension). Tempo three may represent the ideal challenge for you; if not, adjust tempo to a four count to increase intensity. Similarly, if a three count is too difficult, reduce tempo to two. The Spider-Man press-up requires you to alternate each leg for the prescribed repetitions. The rest between sets is displayed as 45–60 seconds (*extend* or *shorten* rest periods specific to your requirements but ensure you take enough rest to replenish the short energy supply). Add or reduce sets to suit requirements.

RESISTANCE STRAIGHT-SETS WORKOUT (ISOTONIC)
Workout 5: Lower Body.
Develop: muscular endurance.
Workout difficulty: 2

Exercise	Reps	Sets	Rest (Between Sets)	Tempo (Count)	Total Workout Time (Approximate)
Wide Squat	15–20	3–4	30–45 Sec	2	
Alternate Lunge	16–20 Alternate Per Leg	3–4	30–45 Sec	2	
Single-Leg RDL	8–10 Per Leg	3–4	30–45 Sec	3	
Calf Raise	15–20	3–4	30–45 Sec	2	
Supine Bridge	15	3–4	30–45 Sec	2	
					15–25 minutes

When using as a standalone workout, include warm-up (five-to-ten minutes), cool-down and stretch (four-to-five minutes). Warm-up time will be specific to your requirements and conditions. Cool-down and stretching time varies and depends on the stretch focus (maintenance or development). Read more on warm-up p.173, cool-down and stretching p.177. Alternatively, filter this workout directly into your existing program (with the assumption that you have already warmed up).

Visual exercise reference

Warm-up exercises	175
Wide Squat	68
Calf Raise	82
Alternate Lunge	73
Supine Bridge	81
Single-Leg RDL	88

Exercise Guide Note: this lower-body resistance workout is targeting a muscular endurance range of 15 – 20 repetitions, representing varying degrees of difficulty, depending on an individual's current strength level. To ensure you remain within the exercise-rep target, adjust your tempo accordingly – slowing the movement down will increase the level of intensity. In this instance, *tempo* has been set at 'two'. This translates to a two count during the concentric phase and the eccentric phase (when the muscles shorten and lengthen under tension). Tempo two may represent the ideal challenge for you; if not, adjust tempo to a three count to increase the intensity. You will notice that the single-leg RDL is set at 'three' already, as the exercise requires this speed to be effective (you can, of course, increase intensity to a 'four'). Also, perform all reps on one leg and then switch to the other (i.e. not alternating). When performing the lunge, alternate legs until 16–20 reps have been completed in total. The rest between sets is displayed as 30–45 seconds (*extend* or *shorten* rest periods specific to your requirements but ensure you take enough rest to replenish the short energy supply). Add or reduce sets to suit requirements.

RESISTANCE STRAIGHT-SETS WORKOUT (ISOTONIC)
Workout 6: Lower Body
Develop: muscular endurance.
Workout difficulty: 2

Exercise	Reps	Sets (Between Sets)	Rest (Count)	Tempo	Total Workout Time (Approximate)
Prisoner Squat	15–20	3–4	30–45 Sec	2	
Side Lunge	16–20 Alternate /Per Leg	3–4	30–45 Sec	2	
Reverse Lunge	16–20 Alternate /Per Leg	3–4	30–45 Sec	2	
Calf Raise	15–20	3–4	30–45 Sec	2	
Donkey Kick to Hip Extension	10 Per Leg	3–4	30–45 Sec	2	
					15–25 Minutes

When using as a standalone workout, include warm-up (five-to-ten minutes), cool-down and stretch (four-to-five minutes). Warm-up time will be specific to your requirements and conditions. Cool-down and stretching time varies and depends on the stretch focus (maintenance or development). Read more on warm-up p.173, cool-down and stretching p.177. Alternatively, filter this workout directly into your existing program (with the assumption that you have already warmed up).

Visual exercise reference

Warm-up exercises	175
Prisoner Squat	69
Calf Raise	82
Side Lunge	75
Donkey Kick to Hip Extension	79
Reverse Lunge	74

This lower-body resistance workout is targeting a muscular endurance range of 15–20 repetitions, representing varying degrees of difficulty depending on an individual's current strength level. To ensure you remain within the exercise-rep target, adjust your tempo accordingly – slowing the movement down will increase the level of intensity. In this instance, *tempo* has been set at 'two'. This translates to a two count during the concentric phase and the eccentric phase (when the muscles shorten and lengthen under tension). Tempo two may represent the ideal challenge for you; if not, adjust tempo to a three count to increase the intensity. When performing both the Side Lunge and Reverse Lunge, alternate legs for the prescribed reps. When performing the Donkey Kick to Hip Extension, complete 10 reps on one leg and then 10 on the other. The rest between sets is displayed as 30–45 seconds (*extend* or *shorten* rest periods specific to your requirements but ensure you take enough rest to replenish the short energy supply). Add or reduce sets to suit requirements.

RESISTANCE STRAIGHT-SETS WORKOUT (ISOTONIC)
Workout 7: Lower Body.
Develop: muscle strength and hypertrophy.
Workout difficulty: 3

Exercise	Reps	Sets	Rest (Between Sets)	Tempo (Count)	Total Workout Time (Approximate)
Bulgarian Squat	8–12 Per leg	3–4	45–60 Sec	2	
Pistol Squat	8–12 Per Leg	3–4	45–60 Sec	2	
Single-Leg RDL	8–12 Per Leg	3–4	45–60 Sec	2	
Single-Leg Bridge	8–12 Per Leg	3–4	45–60 Sec	2	
Calf Raise Single Leg	8–12 Per Leg	3–4	45–60 Sec	2	
					15–25 Minutes

When using as a standalone workout, include warm-up (five-to-ten-minutes), cool-down and stretch (four-to-five minutes). Warm-up time will be specific to your requirements and conditions. Cooldown and stretching time varies and depends on the stretch focus (maintenance or development). Read more on warm-up p.173, cool-down and stretching p.177. Alternatively, filter this workout directly into your existing program (with the assumption that you have already warmed up).

Visual exercise reference

Warm-up exercises	175
Single-Leg Bridge	81
Bulgarian Squat	70
Calf Raise Single Leg	82
Pistol Squat	72
Single-Leg RDL	78

Exercise Guide Note: this lower-body resistance workout is targeting a strength and hypertrophy range of eight to twelve repetitions, representing varying degrees of difficulty depending on an individual's current strength level. To ensure you remain within the exercise target (muscle strength and hypertrophy), adjust your tempo accordingly – slowing the movement down will increase the level of intensity. In this instance, *tempo* has been set at 'two'. This translates to a two count during the concentric phase and the eccentric phase (when the muscles shorten and lengthen under tension). Tempo 'two' may represent the ideal challenge for you; if not, adjust tempo to a three count to increase the intensity. When performing *all* the exercises, complete the prescribed reps for one leg before moving on to the other leg. The rest between sets is displayed as 45–60 seconds (*extend* or *shorten* rest periods specific to your requirements but ensure you take enough rest to replenish the short energy supply). Add or reduce sets to suit requirements.

RESISTANCE ENDURANCE WORKOUT (ISOTONIC)
Workout 8: Chest-shoulder-triceps endurance challenge.
Develop: muscle endurance.
Workout difficulty: 3

Exercise	Reps	Sets	Rest (Between Sets)	Rest (Between Exercises)	Tempo (Count)	Total Work-out Time (Approx)
Standard Press-Up	100>	Mult-iple	As Required	4–5 Mins	2	
Pike Press-Up	100>	Mult-iple	As Required	4–5 Mins	2	
Elevated Dip	100>	Mult-iple	As Required	4–5 Mins	2	
						Variable

When using as a standalone workout, include warm-up (five-to-ten minutes), cool-down and stretch (four-to-five minutes). Warm-up time will be specific to your requirements and conditions. Cool-down and stretching time varies and depends on the stretch focus (maintenance or development). Read more on warm-up p.173, cool-down and stretching p.177. Alternatively, filter this workout directly into your existing program (with the assumption that you have already warmed up).

Visual exercise reference

Warm-up exercises	175
Elevated Dip	63
Standard Press-Up	48
Pike Shoulder Press-Up	57

Exercise Guide Note: this workout should initially be approached as three individual body-part endurance-challenge workouts. There is considerable pre-exhaustion when moving through the exercises, as the triceps are used as synergists (to facilitate movement) in both the standard press-up and pike press-up and then as prime movers with the dips. If you do perform all the exercises in the same workout, take a good rest between exercises. How to approach: perform as many repetitions as you can initially without stopping. As you approach your rep max (the maximum you can perform for that exercise), take a breather – note: do not go to failure, stop several reps short). The length of the rest is your decision; go again as soon as you feel restored (as you become more accustomed, the rests will become shorter). Continue until you reach 100 reps (the > symbol denotes that, if you can complete more, raise the bar!). Take a four-to-five-minute rest between exercises. Perform at a standard tempo 'two'.

RESISTANCE SUPER-SET WORKOUT (ISOTONIC)
Workout 9: Full Body.
Develop: hypertrophy.
Workout difficulty: 4

WORKOUTS AND PROGRAMS

Exercise	Reps	Super Sets	Rest (Between Super Sets)	Tempo (Count)	Total Workout Time (Approximate)
A. Decline Press-Up	12–15		60–90 Sec	2	
		3–4			
B. Pike Shoulder Press-Up	10–12				
A. Diamond Press-Up	10–12	3–4	60–90 Sec	2	
B. Elevated Dip	12–15				
A. Wide Squat	10–12	3–4	60–90 Sec	3	

B. Alternate Lunge	10–12 Per Leg				
A. Bulgarian Squat	8–10 Per Leg	3–4	60–90 Sec	3	
B. Multi-Directional Lunge	10–12 Per Leg				
					16–25 Minutes

When using as a standalone workout, include warm-up (five-to-ten minutes), cool-down and stretch (four-to-five minutes). Warm-up time will be specific to your requirements and conditions. Cool-down and stretching time varies and depends on the stretch focus (maintenance or development). Read more on warm-up p.173, cool-down and stretching p.177. Alternatively, filter this workout directly into your existing program (with the assumption that you have already warmed up).

Visual exercise reference

Wide Squat	68
Pike Shoulder Press-Up	57
Alternate Lunge	73
Diamond Press-up	52
Bulgarian Squat	70

Exercise Guide Note: this full-body resistance super-set workout targets strength and hypertrophy with rep ranges of eight-to-fifteen repetitions. These repetition ranges will represent varying degrees of difficulty, depending on an individual's current strength level. To ensure you remain within the exercise target (muscle strength and hypertrophy), adjust your tempo accordingly – slowing the movement down will increase the level of intensity. In this instance, *tempo for upper-body exercises has been set at 'two'*. This translates to a two count during the concentric phase the eccentric phase (when the muscles shorten and lengthen under tension). Tempo 'two' may represent the ideal challenge for you; if not, adjust tempo to a three count to increase the intensity. *Lower-body exercises have been set at tempo 'three'*. Again, adjust tempo if required to meet reps at the correct intensity. The exercises are grouped together into pairs: perform these groupings as super-sets: **Exercise A (reps)** followed immediately by **Exercise B (reps)** constitutes one *super-set*. Perform three to four super-sets per exercise grouping. Rest between super-sets is 60–90 seconds (*extend* or *shorten* rest periods specific to your requirements but ensure you take enough rest to replenish the short energy supply). Add or reduce sets to suit requirements.

RESISTANCE SUPER-SET WORKOUT (ISOTONIC)

Workout 10: Full Body.
Develop: hypertrophy.
Workout difficulty: 4

Exercise	Reps	Super Sets	Rest (Between Super Sets)	Tempo (Count)	Total Workout Time (Approximate)
A. Dolphin Press-Up	8–10				
		3–4	60–90 Sec	2	
B. Spider-Man Press-Up	10–12				
A. Inch-worm and Press-Up	8–10				
		3–4	60–90 Sec	2	
B. Double Elevated Dip	12–15				

A. Prisoner Squat	10–12				
		3–4	60–90 Sec	3	
B. Wide Squat	10–12 Per Leg				
A. Pistol Squat	6–8 Per Leg				
		3–4	60–90 Sec	3	
B. Calf Raise	15–20				
					16–25 Minutes

When using as a standalone workout, include warm-up (five to ten 10 minutes), cool-down and stretch (four-to-five minutes). Warm-up time will be specific to your requirements and conditions. Cool-down and stretching time varies and depends on the stretch focus (maintenance or development). Read more on warm-up p.173, cool-down and stretching p.177. Alternatively, filter this workout directly into your existing program (with the assumption that you have already warmed up).

Visual exercise reference

Warm-up exercises   175

Exercise Guide Note: this full-body resistance super-set workout targets strength and hypertrophy with rep ranges of eight to fifteen repetitions (exception: 15–20 reps for calf raise). These repetition ranges will represent varying degrees of difficulty, depending on an individual's current strength level. To ensure you remain within the exercise target (muscle strength and hypertrophy), adjust your tempo accordingly – slowing the movement down will increase the level of intensity. In this instance, *tempo for upper-body exercises has been set at 'two'*. This translates to a two count during the concentric phase and the eccentric phase (when the muscles shorten and lengthen under tension). Tempo 'two' may represent the ideal challenge for you; if not, adjust tempo to a three count to increase the intensity. *Lower-body exercises have been set at tempo 'three'*. Again, adjust tempo if required to meet reps at the correct intensity. The exercises are grouped together into pairs: perform these groupings as super-sets. **Exercise A (reps)** followed immediately by **Exercise B (reps)** constitute one *super-set*. Perform three to four super-sets per exercise grouping. Rest between super-sets is 60–90 seconds (*extend* or *shorten* rest periods specific to your requirements but ensure you take enough rest to replenish the short energy supply). Add or reduce sets to suit requirements.

ISOMETRIC (RESISTANCE) WORKOUTS

Read more on isometric exercise on p.30.

Guide

The isometric workouts in this section serve a variety of purposes. Use 'yielding isometrics' for hypertrophy, strength, stability and developing deceleration ability, or for extra ROM with Yielding Eccentric Quasi Isometric (EQI). Use 'overcoming isometrics' for explosive strength, acceleration and ultra-motor-unit-recruitment development. Isometric exercises will also feature in complex workouts.

Frequency: no more than three to four times per week (dependent on other resistance workouts in a given week). Continue to use isometric exercise for no longer than eight weeks, as the adaptation period is quick. Rest for several weeks before resuming.

Equipment

Stopwatch.

Approach

Execute all exercises with proper form, as described. Considerable concentration is required to fully benefit from isometric training. Approach each contraction with 100 per cent focus – what you put in is what you get out. Remember to 'fire' all motor-units when contracting, teaching the body to become more efficient in this process.

Exercise difficulty level

The isometric workouts are all set to variable, as sets, hold and press times/intensity differ greatly from person to person. These workouts are as difficult or as easy as you make them.

Progressions

Progressions can be made through longer holds and presses. Although strength gain and progress is hard to measure with isometrics, rest assured that they are powerful tools to add to your armoury, the benefits of which will be noticeable when performing other types of exercise.

Caution: these programs are not suitable for beginners – a solid fitness background is required before taking part. If you are untrained, sedentary, have underlying health problems or biomechanical issues, it is inadvisable to participate at this level of activity, as there is an increased risk of injury. *If you suffer from high blood pressure, isometric exercises are not advisable.* If in doubt, seek medical advice before attempting any of the workouts.

YIELDING ISOMETRIC CHALLENGE A
Workout 1
Develop: motor-unit recruitment, strength, hypertrophy, stability and ability to decelerate.
Workout difficulty: variable

Exercise	Hold Time	Sets	Fast-and-Loose Drill Between Sets	Rest Between Exercises	Total Workout Time (Approx)
Squat Hold	20–60 Sec	3–5	60 Sec	60–90 Sec	
Press-Up Hold	20–60 Sec	3–5	60 Sec	–	
					8–20 minutes

When using as a standalone workout, include warm-up (five to ten 10 minutes), cool-down and stretch (four-to-five minutes). Warm-up time will be specific to your requirements and conditions. Cool-down and stretching time varies and depends on the stretch focus (maintenance or development). Read more on warm-up p.173, cool-down and stretching p.177. Alternatively, filter this workout directly into your existing program (with the assumption that you have already warmed up).

Visual exercise reference

Warm-up exercises   175
Squat Hold   85
Press-Up Hold   89
Fast-and-Loose Drill
(Either fast and loose uppercuts 107 or fast and loose straight shots 108)

Exercise Guide Note: for those new to isometrics, begin by performing three sets of each exercise for lower time periods – for example, 3 x 30-second squat holds. When progressing, add further sets before you add time. Work towards 5 x 60-second holds (do not exceed a total of 10 minutes' contraction time). If you find yourself able to exceed 60 seconds' holding time, reduce the sets and extend the time. Focus on firing all motor units to maintain position; complete concentration is crucial to progress. Between sets, perform fast-and-loose drills to shake off tension in preparation for the next set. The visual exercise above references two shadow-boxing drills: choose either and perform at a medium intensity. Alternatively, you can perform any exercise or movement that loosens you up. When the squat-hold sets are complete, rest for 60–90 seconds before moving onto the press-up-hold sets. Once the press-up sets are completed, the workout is finished.

YIELDING ISOMETRIC CHALLENGE B
Workout 2
Develop: motor-unit recruitment, strength, hypertrophy, stability and ability to decelerate.
Workout difficulty: variable

Exercise	Hold Time	Sets	Fast-and-Loose Drill Between Sets	Rest Between Exercises	Total Workout Time (Approx)
Lunge Hold	20–60 Per Leg	2–3	60 Sec	60–90 Sec	

Shoulder-Press Hold	20–60 Sec	3–5	60 Sec	–	
					8–20 Minutes

When using as a standalone workout, include warm-up (five-to-ten-minutes), cool-down and stretch (four-to-five minutes). Warm-up time will be specific to your requirements and conditions. Cool-down and stretching time varies and depends on the stretch focus (maintenance or development). Read more on warm-up p.173, cool-down and stretching p.177. Alternatively, filter this workout directly into your existing program (with the assumption that you have already warmed up).

Visual exercise reference

Exercise Guide Note: for those new to isometrics, begin by performing three sets of each exercise for lower time periods – for example, 3 x 30-second lunge holds (note: sets here are two to three per leg).When progressing, add further sets before you add time. Work towards 5 x 60-second holds (do not exceed a total of 10 minutes' contraction time). If you find yourself able to exceed 60 seconds' holding time, reduce the sets and extend the time. Focus on firing all motor units to maintain position; complete concentration is crucial to progress being made. Between sets, perform fast-and-loose drills to shake off tension in preparation for the next set. The visual exercise above references two shadow-boxing drills: choose either and perform at a medium intensity. Alternatively, you can perform any exercise or movement that loosens you up. When the lunge-hold sets are complete, rest for 60–90 seconds before moving onto the pike-press-up-hold sets. Once the latter are completed, the workout is finished.

YIELDING ISOMETRIC CHALLENGE C
Workout 3
Develop: motor-unit recruitment, strength, hypertrophy, stability and ability to decelerate.
Workout difficulty: variable

Exercise	Hold Time	Sets	Fast-and-Loose Drill Between Sets	Rest Between Exercises	Total Workout Time (Approx)
Wall–Squat Hold	45–90 Sec	3–5	60 Sec	60–90 Sec	
Elevated–Dip Hold	20–60 Sec	3–5	60 Sec	–	
					8–20 Minutes

When using as a standalone workout, include warm-up (five-to-ten-minutes), cool-down and stretch (four-to-five minutes). Warm-up time will be specific to your requirements and conditions. Cool-down and stretching time varies and depends on the stretch focus (maintenance or development). Read more on warm-up p.173, cool-down and stretching p.177. Alternatively, filter this workout directly into your existing program (with the assumption that you have already warmed up).

Visual exercise reference

Warm-up exercises	175
Wall-Squat Hold	84
Elevated-Dip Hold	91
Fast-and-Loose Drill	

(Either fast and loose uppercuts 107 or fast and loose straight shots 108)

Exercise Guide Note: for those new to isometrics, begin by performing three sets of each exercise for lower time periods – for example, 3 x 45-second wall-squat holds. When progressing, add further sets before you add time. Work towards 5 x 60-90-second holds (do not exceed a total of 10 minutes' contraction time). If you find yourself able to exceed 60 seconds' holding time, reduce the sets and extend the time. Focus on firing all motor units to maintain position; complete concentration is crucial to progress. Between sets, perform fast-and-loose drills to shake off tension in preparation for the next set. The visual exercise above references two shadow-boxing drills: choose either and perform at medium intensity. Alternatively, you can perform any exercise or movement that loosens you up. When the wall-squat-hold sets are complete, rest for 60–90 seconds before moving onto the elevated-dip-hold sets. Once the latter are completed, the workout is finished.

YIELDING ISOMETRIC CHALLENGE D
Workout 4
Develop: motor-unit recruitment, strength, hypertrophy, stability and ability to decelerate.
Workout difficulty: variable

Exercise	Hold Time	Sets	Fast-and-Loose Drill Between Sets	Rest Between Exercises	Total Workout Time (Approx)
Single-Leg Hold	30–60 Sec per leg	2–3	60 Sec	60–90 Sec	
Single-Leg RDL Hold	20–60 Sec per leg	2–3	60 Sec	–	
					8–20 Minutes

When using as a standalone workout, include warm-up (five-to-ten-minutes), cool-down and stretch (four-to-five minutes). Warm-up time will be specific to your requirements and conditions. Cool-down and stretching time varies and depends on the stretch focus (maintenance or development). Read more on warm-up p.173, cool-

down and stretching p.177. Alternatively, filter this workout directly into your existing program (with the assumption that you have already warmed up).

Visual exercise reference

Warm-up exercises	175
Single-Leg Hold	154
Single-Leg RDL Hold	88
Fast-and-Loose Drill	

(Either fast and loose uppercuts 107 or fast and loose straight shots 108)

Exercise Guide Note: for those new to isometrics, begin by performing three sets of each exercise for lower time periods – for example, 3 x 30-second single-leg holds. When progressing, add further sets before you add time. Work towards 5 x 60-second holds (this workout is set at two to three sets per leg). Do not exceed a total of 10 minutes' contraction time in any one workout. If you find yourself able to exceed 60 seconds' holding time, reduce the sets and extend the time. Focus on firing all motor units to maintain position; complete concentration is crucial to progress being made. Between sets, perform fast-and-loose drills to shake off tension in preparation for the next set. The visual exercise above references two shadow-boxing drills: choose either and perform at medium intensity. Alternatively, you can perform any exercise or movement that loosens you up. When the single-leg-hold sets are complete, rest for 60–90 seconds before moving onto the RDL-hold sets. Once the latter are completed, the workout is finished.

EQI CHALLENGE (YIELDING ISOMETRIC VARIABLE)

Workout 5

Develop: improve motor-unit recruitment, strength, hypertrophy, stability, ability to decelerate and ROM.

Workout difficulty: variable

Exercise	Hold Time	Sets	Fast-and-Loose Drill Between Sets	Rest Between Exercises	Total Workout Time (Approx)
Bulgarian Split Squat EQI	Max Time Per Leg	2–3	60 Sec	60–90 Sec	
Press-up EQI	Max Time	2–3	60 Sec	–	
					8–20 Minutes

When using as a standalone workout, include warm-up (five-to-ten-minutes), cool-down and stretch (four-to-five minutes). Warm-up time will be specific to your requirements and conditions. Cool-down and stretching time varies and depends on the stretch focus (maintenance or development). Read more on warm-up p.173, cool-down and stretching p.177. Alternatively, filter this workout directly into your existing program (with the assumption that you have already warmed up).

Visual exercise reference

Warm-up exercises	175
Bulgarian Split Squat	70
Press-up EQI	48

Fast-and-Loose Drill

(Either fast and loose uppercuts 107 or fast and loose straight shots 108)

Exercise Guide Note: these types of yielding isometrics are called Eccentric Quasi Isometrics (EQIs). Focus on firing all motor units to maintain position – complete concentration is crucial to success. As you fatigue (as time passes), you will sink into the eccentric phase, in doing so increasing your range of movement (ROM) and improving mobility in the end range of a movement. Between sets, perform fast-and-loose drills to shake off tension in preparation for the next set. The visual exercise above references two shadow-boxing drills: choose either and perform at a medium intensity. Alternatively, you can perform any exercise or movement that loosens you up. When Bulgarian-split-squat EQI sets are complete, rest for 60–90 seconds before moving onto the press-up EQI sets. Once the press-up EQI sets are completed, the workout is finished.

OVERCOMING ISOMETRIC A
Workout 6
Develop: ultra-motor-unit recruitment, explosive strength and acceleration.
Workout difficulty: variable

Exercise	Press Time	Sets	Fast-and-Loose Drill Between Sets	Rest Between Exercises	Total Workout Time (Approx)
Wall Shoulder Press	6–10 Sec	3–5	60 Sec	60–90 Sec	
Wall Chest Press	6–10 Sec	3–5	60 Sec	60–90 Sec	
Wall Shoulder Press	6–10 Sec	3–5	60 Sec	–	
					8–20 Minutes

When using as a standalone workout, include warm-up (five-to-ten-minutes), cool-down and stretch (four-to-five minutes). Warm-up time will be specific to your requirements and conditions. Cool-down and stretching time varies and depends on the stretch focus (maintenance or development). Read more on warm-up p.173, cool-down and stretching p.177. Alternatively, filter this workout directly into your existing program (with the assumption that you have already warmed up).

Visual exercise reference
Warm-up exercises   175

Wall Shoulder Press	94
Wall Chest Press	93

Fast and Loose Drill
(Either fast and loose uppercuts 107 or fast and loose straight shots 108)

Exercise Guide Note: this overcoming-isometric workout focuses on improving explosive strength – fast, powerful, explosive movements. When new to this type of training, begin with three sets of six-second contractions (to be executed with full force, with every motor unit fired simultaneously). Over time, increase the sets before increasing the contraction time – work towards five sets of 10-second contractions. Use for no longer than an eight-week period, as the body adapts quickly to isometrics. Take several weeks' break before resuming. Between sets, perform fast-and-loose drills to shake off tension in preparation for the next set. The visual exercise reference above references two shadow-boxing drills: choose either and perform at medium intensity. Alternatively, you can perform any exercise or movement loosens you up.

OVERCOMING ISOMETRIC B/FIGHTER PHASES
Develop: ultra-motor-unit recruitment, explosive strength and acceleration.
Workout difficulty: variable

Exercise	Press Time Per Stage	Sets	Fast-and-Loose Drill Between Sets	Rest Between Exercises	Total Workout Time (Approx)
Jab Three Stages = One Set	6–10 Sec	3–5	60 Sec	60–90 Sec	
Right Cross Three Stages = One Set	6–10 Sec	3–5	60 Sec	–	
					8–20 Mins

When using as a standalone workout, include warm-up (five-to-ten-minutes), cool-down and stretch (four-to-five minutes). Warm-up time will be specific to your requirements and conditions. Cool-down and stretching time varies and depends on the stretch focus (maintenance or development). Read more on warm-up p.173, cool-down and stretching p.177. Alternatively, filter this workout directly into your existing program (with the assumption that you have already warmed up).

Visual exercise reference

(Either fast and loose uppercuts 107 or fast and loose straight shots 108.)

Exercise Guide Note: this overcoming-isometric workout focuses on improving upper-body explosive strength, in particular the three main phases of a boxer's jab and right cross. All three phases should be performed consecutively without a break – this will constitute one set. When new to this type of training, begin with three sets of six-second contractions (to be executed with full force, with every motor unit fired simultaneously). Over time, increase the sets before increasing the contraction time. Work towards five sets of 10-second contractions. Use for no longer than an eight-week period, as the body adapts quickly to isometrics. Take several weeks' break before resuming. Between sets, perform fast-and-loose drills to shake off tension in preparation for the next set. The visual exercise above references two shadow-boxing drills: choose either and perform at medium intensity. Alternatively, you can perform any exercise or movement that loosens you up. When jab sets are complete, rest for 60–90 seconds before moving onto the right-cross sets. Once the right-cross sets have been completed, the workout is finished.

PLYOMETRIC WORKOUTS
Read more on Plyometric exercise on page 27.

Guide
Ensure you have good existing leg strength before engaging in plyometric exercise (specifically the more advanced variations – e.g. depth jumps). If you regularly exercise or are a sportsperson, your existing leg strength should be of a reasonable level to start. However, if new to this kind of explosive training, begin with the lower-medium

level plyometric exercises and gradually work up to the high-level variations as your body becomes more accustomed. Also, start with the lower 'contact' workouts and graduate up. The term 'contact' can be used interchangeably with repetitions but is more commonly used when performing plyometrics due to the nature of the exercise. The prescribed workouts are not rigid; add or reduce sets or contacts to suit your ability. In addition to the cautionary note below, ensure that when performing any depth jumps or box jumps, your chosen elevation is completely secure and stable.

The workouts in this section target speed-strength/power. Particular emphasis is placed on performance-related movement in vertical, horizontal and lateral planes, with focus on improving rate of force. Plyometric exercises will also feature in complex workouts, combined with isometric- and isotonic-resistance components.

Frequency: two to three times per week (dependent on other workouts in a given week; complex workouts, for example – GPP excluded). Three days' rest between workouts is the general recommended recovery period, although 48 hours would suffice. Use these for four to five weeks, then cycle in a rest period of several weeks before resuming. Give the CNS time to recover.

Equipment
Ensure you are wearing cushioned footwear. Avoid performing 'plyos' on concrete surfaces; softer surfaces are less jarring – synthetic, grass, etc.

Approach
Execute all exercises with proper form, as described. Concentrate on *quality*, not *quantity*. We are not concerned with volume: each

repetition/effort should be approached with complete focus on rapid contraction and not on how many repetitions we complete.

Note: conversely, low-level plyometric exercises are used in GPP workouts where the exercise focus is on sustained high-intensity interval training and not on developing the rapid contraction. These more basic exercises work well for GPP, as they facilitate high-intensity regimen.

Exercise difficulty level
The exercise difficulty number indicates how difficult a given workout is.

Progressions
Increase the volume of 'contacts' and sets over time. Progress will manifest in terms of jumping ability (height and distance) and speed strength (how fast and powerfully one can move).

Caution: before engaging in plyometric exercise, you may want to consider an orthopaedic screening to determine if your body can cope with the rigours of this type of impact exercise. These programs are not suitable for beginners – a solid fitness background is required before taking part. If you are untrained, sedentary, have underlying health problems or biomechanical issues, it is inadvisable to participate at this level of activity, as there is an increased risk of injury. If in doubt, seek medical advice before attempting any of the workouts.

PLYOMETRIC CONTACT 60
Workout 1
Develop: upper-body explosive strength and vertical-jump height.
Workout difficulty: 1 (targets those with lower upper-body strength)

Exercise	Contacts	Sets	Rest Between Sets	Total Workout Time (Approx)
Extended-Kneeling Plyometric Press-Up	8-10	3	60-90 Sec	
Tuck Jump	8-10	3	60-90 Sec	
				7-10 Minutes

When using as a standalone workout, include warm-up (five-to-ten-minutes), cool-down and stretch (four-to-five minutes). Warm-up time will be specific to your requirements and conditions. Cool-down and stretching time varies and depends on the stretch focus (maintenance or development). Read more on warm-up p.173, cool-down and stretching p.177. Alternatively, filter this workout directly into your existing program (with the assumption that you have already warmed up).

Visual exercise reference

Exercise Guide Note: this workout is aimed at those new to plyometric exercise and is called Contact 60, as it involves 6 x 10 contacts in total. With both exercises, take a pause between each repetition as opposed to working continuously (this will come later). Focus on rapid contraction in each repetition. Rest for 60–90 seconds between each set, giving your CNS a rest. Once all the sets of one exercise are complete, move onto the next exercise.

Experiment by exchanging the exercises: e.g. swap vertical jump for another standing jump: lunge jump, squat jump or frog jump. Remember that, for this workout, reps are performed with pauses – i.e. not continuously.

PLYOMETRIC CONTACT 60

Workout 2

Develop: upper-body explosive strength and vertical jump height.

Workout difficulty: 1

Exercise	Contacts	Sets	Rest Between Sets	Total Workout Time (Approx)
Hand–Clap Plyometric Press-Up	10	3	60–90 Sec	
Squat Jump	10	3	60–90 Sec	
				7–10 Minutes

When using as a standalone workout, include warm-up (five-to-ten-minutes), cool-down and stretch (four-to-five minutes). Warm-up time will be specific to your requirements and conditions. Cool-down and stretching time varies and depends on the stretch focus (maintenance or development). Read more on warm-up p.173, cool-down and stretching p.177. Alternatively, filter this workout directly into your existing program (with the assumption that you have already warmed up).

Visual exercise reference

Warm-up exercises	175
Hand-Clap Plyometric Press-Up	100
Squat Jump	113

Exercise Guide Note: this workout is aimed at those new to plyometric exercise and is called Contact 60, as it involves 6 x 10 contacts in total. With both exercises, take a pause between each repetition as opposed to working continuously (this will come later). Focus on rapid contraction in each repetition. Rest for 60–90 seconds between each set, giving your CNS a rest. Once all the sets of one exercise are complete, move onto the next exercise.

Experiment by exchanging the exercises: e.g. swap vertical jump for another standing jump: lunge jump, squat jump or frog jump. Remember that, for this workout, reps are performed with pauses – i.e. not continuously.

PLYOMETRIC CONTACT 90
Workout 3
Develop: vertical and horizontal power and improved deceleration.
Workout difficulty: 2

Exercise	Contacts	Sets	Rest Between Sets	Total Workout Time (Approx)
Standing Vertical Jump	8	3	60–90 Sec	
Forward Single-Leg Hop	6 Per Leg	3	60–90 Sec	
Standing Long Jump	10	3	60–90 Sec	
				10–15 Minutes

When using as a standalone workout, include warm-up (five-to-ten-minutes), cool-down and stretch (four-to-five minutes). Warm-up time will be specific to your requirements and conditions. Cool-down and stretching time varies and depends on the stretch focus (maintenance or development). Read more on warm-up p.173, cool-down and stretching p.177. Alternatively, filter this workout directly into your existing program (with the assumption that you have already warmed up).

Visual exercise reference

Forward Single-leg Hop   129

Standing Long Jump   128

Exercise Guide Note: this workout represents a medium-level plyometric workout, great for developing horizontal power for sprinting-based sports, also adding a vertical-jump component to increase vertical-jump height and forward single-leg hops, developing horizontal power and deceleration (ability to stop quickly – as in basketball and football). Focus is on rapid contraction in each repetition. Perform vertical jump continuously; the single-leg hop and standing long jump are executed with a pause, to reset before you execute another repetition. Rest for 60–90 seconds between each set, giving your CNS a rest. Once all the sets of one exercise are complete, move onto the next exercise.

PLYOMETRIC CONTACT 90
Workout 4
Develop: vertical power.
Workout difficulty: 2

Exercise	Contacts	Sets	Rest Between Sets	Total Workout Time (Approx)
Ankle Jump	10	3	60–90 Sec	
Squat Jump	10	3	60–90 Sec	

Tuck Jump	10	3	60–90 Sec	
				10–15 minutes

When using as a standalone workout, include warm-up (five-to-ten-minutes), cool-down and stretch (four-to-five minutes). Warm-up time will be specific to your requirements and conditions. Cool-down and stretching time varies and depends on the stretch focus (maintenance or development). Read more on warm-up p.173, cool-down and stretching p.177. Alternatively, filter this workout directly into your existing program (with the assumption that you have already warmed up).

Visual exercise reference

Warm-up exercises	175
Ankle Jump	119
Squat Jump	113
Tuck Jump	111

Exercise Guide Note: this workout represents a medium-level plyometric workout with the specific aim of improving vertical power. Perform all exercises continuously for the prescribed repetitions. Focus on rapid contraction in each repetition. Rest for 60–90 seconds between each set, giving your CNS a rest. Once all the sets of one exercise are complete, move onto the next exercise.

'THE FOOTBALLER' – PLYOMETRIC CONTACT 110
Workout 5
Develop: horizontal power and improved deceleration.
Workout difficulty: 3

Exercise	Contacts	Sets	Rest Between Sets	Total Workout Time (Approx)
Multiple Standing Long Jumps	5	4	90–120 Sec	
Lateral Single-Leg Hop	5 per leg	3	90–120 Sec	
Forward-and-Back Single-Leg Hop	10 per leg	3	90–120 Sec	
				12–15 minutes

When using as a standalone workout, include warm-up (five-to-ten-minutes), cool-down and stretch (four-to-five minutes). Warm-up time will be specific to your requirements and conditions. Cool-down and stretching time varies and depends on the stretch focus (maintenance or development). Read more on warm-up p.173, cool-

down and stretching p.177. Alternatively, filter this workout directly into your existing program (with the assumption that you have already warmed up).

Visual exercise reference

Exercise Guide Note: 'The Footballer' represents a medium-level plyometric workout. The concentration here is on developing horizontal (sprinting) power, deceleration (stopping quickly) and focusing on ankle and hip stability, particularly useful for footballers. Other sports that involve stop-start characteristics will benefit greatly from the workout, as well as improving deceleration capabilities. Focus on rapid contraction in each repetition. Multiple standing long jumps are as described, lateral single-leg hops have a stabilising component (for deceleration), as per description, forward-and-back single-leg hops are performed continuously. Rest for 90–120 seconds between each set, giving your CNS a rest. Once all the sets of one exercise are complete, move onto the next exercise.

'THE ALL-ROUNDER' – PLYOMETRIC CONTACT 140
Workout 6
Develop: multi-directional power and improved deceleration.
Workout difficulty: 3

Exercise	Contacts	Sets	Rest Between Sets	Total Workout Time (Approx)
Forward Bounds	5	4	90–120 Sec	
45-Degree Single-Leg Hop	5 per leg	3	90–120 Sec	
Hop, Skip and Jump	5 Cycles Per Leg	3	90–120 Sec	
				12–15 minutes

When using as a standalone workout, include warm-up (five-to-ten-minutes), cool-down and stretch (four-to-five minutes). Warm-up time will be specific to your requirements and conditions. Cool-down and stretching time varies and depends on the stretch focus (maintenance or development). Read more on warm-up p.173, cool-down and stretching p.177. Alternatively, filter this workout directly into your existing program (with the assumption that you have already warmed up).

Visual exercise reference

Exercise Guide Note: 'The All-Rounder' represents a medium-high-level plyometric workout. The concentration here is on developing multi-directional power for all-round performance. Focus on rapid contraction in each repetition. Forward bounds are performed continuously for 6 bounds, followed by the 45-degree single-leg hop that has a stabilising component (for deceleration), as per description, and lastly hop, skip and jump is performed in a three-contact phase with a pause between each cycle. Rest for 90-120 seconds between each set, giving your CNS a break. Once all the sets of one exercise are complete, move onto the next exercise.

Note: Hop, Skip and Jump is denoted in cycles: this is due to the exercise being in three-contact phases, which will equal one cycle. Perform three sets of five cycles per leg, computing to 90 contacts.

'THE BASKETBALLER' – PLYOMETRIC CONTACT 129
Workout 7
Develop: multi-directional power and improved deceleration.
Workout difficulty: 3

Exercise	Contacts	Sets	Rest Between Sets	Total Workout Time (Approx)
Ankle Jump	10	3	90–120 Sec	
Vertical Jump	8	3	90–120 Sec	
Multiple Standing Long Jump	5	3	90–120 Sec	
Side-to-Side Single-Leg Hop	10 per leg	3	90–120 Sec	
				15–20 Minutes

When using as a standalone workout, include warm-up (five-to-ten-minutes), cool-down and stretch (four-to-five minutes). Warm-up time will be specific to your requirements and conditions. Cool-down and stretching time varies and depends on the stretch focus (maintenance or development). Read more on warm-up p.273, cool-down and stretching p.277. Alternatively, filter this workout directly into your existing program (with the assumption that you have already warmed up).

Visual exercise reference

Exercise Guide Note: 'The Basketballer' represents a medium-high level plyometric workout and mainly focuses on vertical-jump strength. Focus on rapid contraction in each repetition. The ankle jumps should be performed in a continuous fast action. All exercises are performed as continuous. Rest for 90–120 seconds between each set, giving your CNS a break. Once all the sets of one exercise are complete, move onto the next exercise.

'THE SPRINTER' – PLYOMETRIC CONTACT 100
Workout 8
Develop: horizontal power.
Workout difficulty: 3

Exercise	Contacts	Sets	Rest Between Sets	Total Workout Time (Approx)
Depth Jump to Standing Long Jump	5	5	90–120 Sec	
Forward Bounds	10	5	90–120 Sec	

Multiple Standing Long Jump	5	5	90–120 Sec	
				15–20 minutes

When using as a standalone workout, include warm-up (five-to-ten-minutes), cool-down and stretch (four-to-five minutes). Warm-up time will be specific to your requirements and conditions. Cool-down and stretching time varies and depends on the stretch focus (maintenance or development). Read more on warm-up – XX, cool-down and stretching – XX. Alternatively, filter this workout directly into your existing program (with the assumption that you have already warmed up).

Visual exercise reference

Exercise Guide Note: 'The Sprinter' represents a high-level plyometric workout and mainly focuses on horizontal power. Focus on rapid contraction in each repetition. The depth jump to standing long jump is per exercise description; bounds and multiple long jumps are continuous. Rest for 90–120 seconds between each set, giving your CNS a break. Once all the sets of one exercise are complete, move onto the next exercise.

'THE FIGHTER' – PLYOMETRIC CONTACT 90

Workout 9
Develop: upper-body, vertical and horizontal power.
Workout difficulty: 4

Exercise	Contacts	Sets	Rest Between Sets	Total Workout Time (Approx)
Full-Body Plyometric Press-Up	8-10	3	90-120 Sec	
Squat Jump	10	3	90-120 Sec	
Kneeling Jump to Squat Hold	10	3	90-120 Sec	
				10-15 minutes

When using as a standalone workout, include warm-up (five-to-ten-minutes), cool-down and stretch (four-to-five minutes). Warm-up time will be specific to your requirements and conditions. Cool-down and stretching time varies and depends on the stretch focus (maintenance or development). Read more on warm-up p.173, cool-down and stretching p.177. Alternatively, filter this workout directly into your existing program (with the assumption that you have already warmed up).

Visual exercise reference

Exercise Guide Note: 'The Fighter' represents a high-intensity plyometric workout, with two of the components being ultra-high intensity. The focus here is on building upper-body power along with vertical and horizontal power (explosive hip and leg power is integral to throwing powerful punches). The full-body plyometric press-up should be performed continuously, as with the squat jump; the kneeling jump to squat hold will involve a pause in the squat before executing the next repetition. Rest for 90–120 seconds between each set, giving your CNS a break. Once all the sets of one exercise are complete, move onto the next exercise.

'THE POWER-UP' – PLYOMETRIC CONTACT 85
Workout 10
Develop: upper-body, vertical and horizontal power.
Workout difficulty: 4

Exercise	Contacts	Sets	Rest Between Sets	Total Workout Time (Approx)
Chest-Slap Plyometric Press-Up	8-10	3	90–120 Sec	

Tuck Jump	10	3	90–120 Sec	
Depth Jump to Vertical Jump	5	5	90–120 Sec	
				12–15 Minutes

When using as a standalone workout, include warm-up (five-to-ten-minutes), cool-down and stretch (four-to-five minutes). Warm-up time will be specific to your requirements and conditions. Cool-down and stretching time varies and depends on the stretch focus (maintenance or development). Read more on warm-up p.173, cool-down and stretching p.177. Alternatively, filter this workout directly into your existing program (with the assumption that you have already warmed up).

Visual exercise reference

Exercise Guide Note: 'The Power-Up' represents a high-intensity plyometric workout, with one of the components being ultra-high intensity. The focus here is on building upper-body power along with vertical power. The chest-slap plyometric press-up should be performed continuously, as with the tuck jump; the depth jump to vertical jump will involve a reset to position before executing the next repetition. Rest for 90–120 seconds between each set, giving your CNS a break. Once all the sets of one exercise are complete, move onto the next exercise.

COMPLEX WORKOUTS
Read more on complex exercise on page 35.

Guide
The complex workouts in this section represent the gold standard in terms of explosive-strength development. They combine both isotonic and isometric resistance exercises with plyometric exercises, researched as the optimum combinations in developing rate of force. Read more on complex training on page 35. These workouts require a high capacity, so approach with care. Ensure you have good existing leg strength before engaging in plyometric exercise (specifically the more advanced variations – e.g. depth jumps). If you regularly exercise or are a sportsperson, your existing leg strength should be of a reasonable level to start. However, if new to this kind of explosive training, begin with the lower-medium level plyometric exercises and gradually work up to the high-level variations as your body becomes more accustomed. The prescribed workouts are not rigid; add or reduce sets, repetitions or contacts to suit your level of ability. As you become more accustomed to the workouts, experiment by exchanging exercises. In addition to the cautionary note below, ensure that when performing any depth jumps or box jumps, your chosen elevation is completely secure and stable.

Frequency: one to two times per week (dependent on other workouts in any given week), with 48 hours' rest between workouts. Use these for four to five weeks, then cycle in a rest period of several weeks before resuming. Give the CNS time to recover.

Equipment
Ensure you are wearing cushioned footwear. Avoid performing plyometrics on concrete surfaces; softer surfaces are less jarring – synthetic, grass, etc.

Approach
Execute all exercises with proper form, as described. Concentrate on *quality*, not *quantity*. We are not concerned with volume; each repetition/effort of the plyometric component should be approached with complete focus on rapid contraction.

Exercise difficulty level
The exercise-difficulty number indicates how difficult a given workout is.

Progressions
Make progressions in variety of ways: add reps and sets; decrease tempo for resistance repetitions; increase time for yielding isometrics, refining and improving explosiveness when executing plyometric and overcoming-isometric exercises.

Caution: before engaging in plyometric exercise, you may want to consider an orthopaedic screening to determine whether your body can cope with the rigours of this type of impact exercise. These programs are not suitable for beginners – a solid fitness background is required before taking part. If you are untrained, sedentary, have underlying health problems or biomechanical issues, it is inadvisable to participate at this level of activity, as there is an increased risk of injury. If in doubt, seek medical advice before attempting any of the workouts.

COMPLEX CHALLENGE 1 (USING ISOTONIC RESISTANCE AND PLYOMETRIC COMBINATION)

Workout 1
Develop: explosive strength.
Workout difficulty: 2

Exercise	Repetitions	Sets	Count/ Speed	Rest Between Sets	Total Workout Time (Approx)
Standard Squat	10–12	3	3	45–60 Sec	
Alternate Lunge	10–12 Per Leg	3	3	45–60 Sec	
Standard Press-Up	10–12	3	3	45–60 Sec	
Squat Jump	8–10	3	Rapid	60–90 Sec	
Tuck Jump	8–10	3	Rapid	60–90 Sec	
Hand-Clap Plyometric Press-Up	8–10	3	Rapid	60–90 Sec	
					Variable

When using as a standalone workout, include warm-up (five-to-ten-minutes), cool-down and stretch (four-to-five minutes). Warm-up time will be specific to your requirements and conditions. Cool-down and stretching time varies and depends on the stretch focus (maintenance or development). Read more on warm-up p.173, cool-down and stretching p.177. Alternatively, filter this workout directly into your existing program (with the assumption that you have already warmed up).

Visual exercise reference

Warm-up exercises	175
Squat Jump	113
Standard Squat	66
Tuck Jump	111
Alternate Lunge	73
Hand-Clap Plyometric Press-Up	100
Standard Press-Up	48

Exercise Guide Note: perform all exercises consecutively. Begin with the first three resistance exercises. Aim to complete 10–12 reps, adjusting the count to fit your ability. The number count represents the numbers you count concentrically (when muscle shortens) and eccentrically (when muscle lengthens). Therefore, a 'three' is more intense than a 'two', as the muscles are under tension for longer; a 'four' would constitute even more intensity. Set your level so that 10–12 reps becomes challenging. Rest between sets as prescribed, or adjust according to your needs. Once you have completed the resistance component, move onto the plyometric component. All plyometric repetitions (contacts) should be executed rapidly and continuously. Take adequate rest between sets and exercises as prescribed, giving your CNS time to recover.

COMPLEX CHALLENGE 2 (USING ISOTONIC RESISTANCE AND PLYOMETRIC COMBINATION)

Workout 2

Develop: explosive strength.

Workout difficulty: 2

Exercise	Repetitions	Sets	Count/ Speed	Rest Between Sets	Total Workout Time (Approx)
Wide Squat	10–12	3	3	45–60 Sec	
Side Lunge	10–12 Per Leg	3	3	45–60 Sec	
Decline Press-Up	10–12	3	3	45–60 Sec	
Ankle Jump	8–10	3	Rapid	60–90 Sec	
Lunge Jump	8–10	3	Rapid	60–90 Sec	
Chest-Slap Plyometric Press-Up	8–10	3	Rapid	60–90 Sec	
					Variable

When using as a standalone workout, include warm-up (five-to-ten-minutes), cool-down and stretch (four-to-five minutes). Warm-up time will be specific to your requirements and conditions. Cool-down and stretching time varies and depends on the stretch focus (maintenance or development). Read more on warm-up p.173, cool-down and stretching p.177. Alternatively, filter this workout directly into your existing program (with the assumption that you have already warmed up).

Visual exercise reference

Warm-up exercises	175
Ankle Jump	119
Wide Squat	68
Lunge Jump	118
Side Lunge	75
Chest-Slap Plyometric Press-Up	102
Decline Press-Up	57

Exercise Guide Note: perform all exercises consecutively. Begin with the first three resistance exercises. Aim to complete 10–12 reps, adjusting the count to fit your ability. The number count represents the numbers you count concentrically (when muscle shortens) and eccentrically (when muscle lengthens). Therefore, a 'three' is more intense than a 'two', as the muscles are under tension for longer; a 'four' would constitute even more intensity. Set your level so that 10-12 reps becomes challenging. Rest between sets as prescribed, or adjust according to your needs. Once you have completed the resistance component, move onto the plyometric component. All plyometric repetitions (contacts) should be executed rapidly and continuously. Take adequate rest between sets and exercises as prescribed, giving your CNS time to recover.

COMPLEX SUPER-SET CHALLENGE 3 (USING ISOTONIC RESISTANCE AND PLYOMETRIC COMBINATION)

Workout 3

Develop: explosive strength.

Workout difficulty: 3

Exercise	Super-Sets	Repetitions	Count/Speed	Rest Between Sets	Total Workout Time (Approx)
Standard Squat	3	10–12	3	2–3 Mins	
Standing Long Jump		8	Rapid		
Pike Shoulder Press-up	3	10–12	3	2–3 Mins	
Hand-Clap Plyometric Press-Up		8	Rapid		
Calf Raise	3	12–15	3	2–3 Mins	
Ankle Jump		8	Rapid		
					Variable

When using as a standalone workout, include warm-up (five-to-ten-minutes), cool-down and stretch (four-to-five minutes). Warm-up time will be specific to your requirements and conditions. Cool-down and stretching time varies and depends on the stretch focus (maintenance or development). Read more on warm-up p.173, cool-down and stretching p.177. Alternatively, filter this workout directly into your existing program (with the assumption that you have already warmed up).

Visual exercise reference

Warm-up exercises	175
Hand-Clap Plyometric Press-Up	100
Standard Squat	66
Calf Raise	82
Standing Long Jump	128
Ankle Jump	119
Pike Shoulder Press-Up	57

Exercise Guide Note: this super-set challenge captures the principles of pure complex training by preparing and making available the fast-twitch fibres for the immediate ensuing plyometric stimulus, maximising the rate of force potential. There are three pairs of exercises to be performed as three super-sets per pair. For example, begin by performing the standard squat – one set of 10–12 reps – immediately followed by standing long jumps (perform these rapidly and in singles, not continuously): one set x eight reps. This will constitute one super-set. Complete two more super-sets for that pairing, then move onto the next pairing. Plyometric press-up and ankle-jump reps are performed continuously without stopping. Rest for two-to-three minutes between supersets.

Note: The number count represents the numbers you count concentrically (when the muscle shortens) and eccentrically (when the muscle lengthens). Therefore, a 'three' is more intense than a 'two', as the muscles are under tension for longer; a 'four' would constitute even more intensity. Set your level so that 10–12 reps becomes challenging. Rest between sets as prescribed, or adjust according to your needs.

COMPLEX SUPER-SET CHALLENGE 4 (USING ISOTONIC RESISTANCE AND PLYOMETRIC COMBINATION)

Workout 4

Develop: explosive strength.

Workout difficulty: 3

Exercise	Super-Sets	Repetitions	Count/Speed	Rest Between Sets	Total Workout Time (Approx)
Prisoner Squat	3	10–12	3	2–3 Mins	
Depth Jump to Standing Long Jump		5	Rapid		
Decline Press-Up	3	10–12	3	2–3 Mins	
Hand-Clap Plyometric Press-up		8	Rapid		

Wide Squat	3	10–12	3	2–3 Mins	
Frog Jump		8	Rapid		
					Variable

When using as a standalone workout, include warm-up (five-to-ten-minutes), cool-down and stretch (four-to-five minutes). Warm-up time will be specific to your requirements and conditions. Cool-down and stretching time varies and depends on the stretch focus (maintenance or development). Read more on warm-up p.173, cool-down and stretching p.177. Alternatively, filter this workout directly into your existing program (with the assumption that you have already warmed up).

Visual exercise reference

Warm-up exercises	175
Hand-Clap Plyometric Press-Up	100
Prisoner Squat	69
Wide Squat	68
Depth Jump to Standing Long Jump	140
Frog Jump	116
(Try Box Jump if solid elevation available 138)	
Decline Press-Up	57

Exercise Guide Note: this super-set challenge captures the principles of pure complex training by preparing and making available the fast-twitch fibres for the immediate ensuing plyometric stimulus, maximising rate of force potential. There are three pairs of exercises to be performed as three super-sets per pair. For example, begin by performing prisoner squat – one set of 10–12 reps – immediately followed by depth jump to standing long jump (perform these rapidly and in singles, not continuously) – one set x five reps. This will constitute one super-set. Complete two more super-sets for that pairing, then move onto the next. Plyometric press-up and ankle-jump reps are performed continuously without stopping. Rest for two to three minutes between super-sets.

Note: The number count represents the numbers you count concentrically (when the muscle shortens) and eccentrically (when the muscle lengthens). Therefore, a 'three' is more intense than a 'two', as the muscles are under tension for longer; a 'four' would constitute even more intensity. Set your level so that 10–12 reps becomes challenging. Rest between sets as prescribed, or adjust according to your needs.

COMPLEX SUPER-SET CHALLENGE 5 (USING YIELDING ISOMETRIC RESISTANCE AND PLYOMETRIC COMBINATION)
Workout 5
Develop: explosive strength.
Workout difficulty: 4

Exercise	Super-Sets	Repetitions	Count/Speed	Rest Between Sets	Total Workout Time (Approx)
Squat Hold (Yielding Isometric)	3	One hold	20–40 Sec	2–3 Mins	
Squat Jump		8	Rapid		
Press-Up Hold (Yielding Isometric)	3	One hold	20–40 Secs	2–3 Mins	
Hand-Clap Plyometric Press-Up		8	Rapid		
Single-Leg Hold (Yielding Isometric)	3	One hold	20–40 Sec per leg	2–3 Mins	
Forward-and-Back Single-Leg Hop		8 per leg	Rapid		
					Variable

When using as a standalone workout, include warm-up (five-to-ten-minutes), cool-down and stretch (four-to-five minutes). Warm-up time will be specific to your requirements and conditions. Cool-down and stretching time varies and depends on the stretch focus (maintenance or development). Read more on warm-up p.173, cool-down and stretching p.177. Alternatively, filter this workout directly into your existing program (with the assumption that you have already warmed up).

Visual exercise reference

Warm-up exercises	175
Hand-Clap Plyometric Press-Up	100
Squat Hold	85
Single-Leg Hold	154
Squat Jump	113
Forward-and-Back Single-Leg Hop	134
Press-Up Hold	89

Exercise Guide Note: this super-set challenge captures the principles of pure complex training by preparing and making available the fast-twitch fibres using yielding isometrics (fire all motor units to maintain position) for the immediate ensuing plyometric stimulus, maximising rate-of-force potential. There are three pairs of exercises to be performed as three super-sets per pair. For example, begin by performing the squat hold for a time (20–40 seconds), immediately followed by the squat jump. Execute these continuously for one set x eight reps. This will constitute one super-set. Complete two more super-sets for that pairing, then move onto the next pairing. All plyometric components are performed continuously without stopping. Rest for two to three minutes between super-sets.

COMPLEX SUPER-SET CHALLENGE 6 (USING OVERCOMING ISOMETRIC RESISTANCE AND PLYOMETRIC COMBINATION)

Workout 6

Develop: explosive strength.

Workout difficulty: 4

Exercise	Super-Sets	Repetitions	Count/ Speed	Rest Between Sets	Total Workout Time (Approx)
Wall Chest Press (Over-coming Isometric)	4	One hold	6–10 Sec	2–3 Mins	
Hand-Clap Plyometric Press-Up		8	Rapid		
Wall Shoulder Press (Over-coming Isometric)	4	One hold	6–10 Sec	2–3 Mins	
Full-body Plyometric Press-Up		6-8	Rapid		
					Variable

When using as a standalone workout, include warm-up (five-to-ten-minutes), cool-down and stretch (four-to-five minutes). Warm-up time will be specific to your requirements and conditions. Cool-down and stretching time varies and depends on the stretch focus (maintenance or development). Read more on warm-up p.173, cool-down and stretching p.177. Alternatively, filter this workout directly into your existing program (with the assumption that you have already warmed up).

Visual exercise reference

Warm-up exercises	175
Wall Chest Press	93
Wall Shoulder Press	94
Hand-Clap Plyometric Press-Up	100
Full-Body Plyometric Press-Up	103

Exercise Guide Note: this super-set challenge captures the principles of pure complex training by preparing and making available the fast-twitch fibres using overcoming isometrics (approach these with 100 per cent intensity, total motor-unit activation pressing as hard and as fast as possible) for the immediate ensuing plyometric stimulus, maximising rate-of-force potential. There are two pairs of exercises to be performed as four super-sets per pair. For example, begin by performing the wall chest press for a time (six to ten seconds), immediately followed by the hand-clap plyometric press-up. Execute these continuously for one x eight reps. This will constitute one super-set. Complete three more super-sets for that pairing, then move onto the next. All plyometric components are performed continuously without stopping. Rest for two to three minutes between super-sets.

ADVANCED COMPLEX SUPER-SET CHALLENGE 7 (USING ISOTONIC RESISTANCE AND PLYOMETRIC COMBINATION)

Workout 7

Develop: explosive strength.

Workout difficulty: 4

Exercise	Super-Sets	Repetitions	Count/Speed	Rest Between Sets	Total Workout Time (Approx)
Pistol Squat	3	6-8 per leg	3	2-3 Mins	
Multiple Standing Long Jump		5	Rapid		
Spider-Man Press-Up	3	6-8 alternate legs	3	2-3 Mins	
Full-Body Plyometric Press-Up		6-8	Rapid		
Single-Leg RDL	3	6-8 per leg	3	2-3 Mins	
Depth Jump to Vertical Jump		5	Rapid		
					Variable

When using as a standalone workout, include warm-up (five-to-ten-minutes), cool-down and stretch (four-to-five minutes). Warm-up time will be specific to your requirements and conditions. Cool-down and stretching time varies and depends on the stretch focus (maintenance or development). Read more on warm-up p.173, cool-down and stretching p.177. Alternatively, filter this workout directly into your existing program (with the assumption that you have already warmed up).

Visual exercise reference

Warm-up exercises	175
Full-Body Plyometric Press-up	103
Pistol Squat	72
Single-Leg RDL	78
Multiple Standing Long Jump	143
Depth Jump to Vertical Jump	140
Spider-Man Press-Up	53

Exercise Guide Note: this advanced super-set challenge captures the principles of pure complex training by preparing and making available the fast-twitch fibres for the immediate ensuing plyometric stimulus, maximising rate-of-force potential. There are three pairs of exercises to be performed as three super-sets per pair. For example, begin by performing the pistol squat (any variation) – one set x six to eight reps per leg – immediately followed by the multiple standing long jump – one set x five reps. This will constitute one super-set. Complete two more super-sets for that pairing, then move onto the next pairing. Full-body plyometric press-up reps should be performed continuously without stopping. The depth jump to vertical jump should be performed in single rapid contractions for the prescribed reps. Rest for two to three minutes between supersets.

Note: The number count represents the numbers you count concentrically (when the muscle shortens) and eccentrically (when the muscle lengthens). Therefore, a 'three' is more intense than a 'two', as the muscles are under tension for longer; a 'four' would constitute even more intensity. Set your level so that six to eight reps becomes challenging. Rest between sets, as prescribed, or adjust according to your needs.

ADVANCED COMPLEX SUPER-SET CHALLENGE 8 (USING ISOTONIC RESISTANCE AND PLYOMETRIC COMBINATION)

Workout 8

Develop: explosive strength.

Workout difficulty: 4

Exercise	Super-Sets	Repetitions	Count/Speed	Rest Between Sets	Total Workout Time (Approx)
Standard Squat	3	10–12	3	2–3 Mins	
Standing Vertical Jump		8	Rapid		
Decline Pike Shoulder Press-Up	3	10–12	3	2–3 Mins	

Chest-Slap Plyometric Press-Up		8	Rapid		
Bulgarian Squat	3	8 per leg	3	2–3 Mins	
Side-to-Side Single-Leg Hop		10 per per leg	Rapid		
					Variable

When using as a standalone workout, include warm-up (five-to-ten-minutes), cool-down and stretch (four-to-five minutes). Warm-up time will be specific to your requirements and conditions. Cool-down and stretching time varies and depends on the stretch focus (maintenance or development). Read more on warm-up p.173, cool-down and stretching p.177. Alternatively, filter this workout directly into your existing program (with the assumption that you have already warmed up).

Visual exercise reference

Exercise Guide Note: this advanced super-set complex challenge captures the principles of pure complex training by preparing and making available the fast-twitch fibres for the immediate ensuing plyometric stimulus, maximising rate-of-force potential. There are three pairs of exercises to be performed as three super-sets per pair. For example, begin by performing the standard squat – one set of 10–12 – immediately followed by the standing vertical jump – one set x eight reps. This will constitute one super-set. Complete two more super-sets for that pairing, then move onto the next pairing. Chest-slap plyometric press-up reps and side-to-side single-leg hops should be performed continuously without stopping. Rest for two-to-three minutes between supersets.

Note: The number count represents the numbers you count concentrically (when the muscle shortens) and eccentrically (when the muscle lengthens). Therefore, a 'three' is more intense than a 'two', as the muscles are under tension for longer; a 'four' would constitute even more intensity. Set your level so that 10–12 reps becomes challenging. Rest between sets, as prescribed, or adjust according to your needs.

CORE WORKOUTS

Read more on core workouts on page 37.

Guide

This section provides *direct* targeting of the core muscles with repetition and timed workouts. However, virtually all of the bodyweight exercises in this book use the core muscles to stabilise and initiate movement, as they are functional by nature. Use these core workouts as an opportunity to gain muscle awareness and control over the inner and outer units of the trunk, then carry this skill and improved core stability into your exercises.

Frequency: this is open to debate: as we use and engage the core on a daily basis, we should, in theory, benefit from direct training on the same basis. However, two to three times per week is perfectly sufficient.

Equipment

A stopwatch is required for the timed workouts.

Approach

Pay special attention to engaging the correct muscles in contraction; build awareness around your body.

Workout difficulty level

Each workout has a difficulty number; the higher the number, the more challenging the workout. Be creative and experiment using alternative exercises from the Exercise Portfolio.

Progressions

Focus on correct application, especially when engaging the transverse abdominis. Strive to develop both the inner and outer units of the trunk into one powerful mechanism.

Caution: these programs are not suitable for beginners – a solid fitness background is required before taking part. If you are untrained, sedentary, have underlying health problems or biomechanical issues, it is inadvisable to participate at this level of activity, as there is an increased risk of injury. If in doubt, seek medical advice before attempting any of the workouts.

CORE WORKOUT – REPETITION CIRCUITS
Workout 1
Workout difficulty: 2

Exercise	Reps	Circuits
Side Plank with Twist	8–10 per side	
Bird Dog	6–8 per side	
Seated Row Crunch	15–20	
Alternate Crunch	8–10 per side	
Reverse Curl	8–10	
1 Circuit		2–3

When using as a standalone workout, include warm-up (five-to-ten-minutes), cool-down and stretch (four-to-five minutes). Warm-up time will be specific to your requirements and conditions. Cool-down and stretching time varies and depends on the stretch focus (maintenance or development). Read more on warm-up p.173, cool-down and stretching p.177. Alternatively, filter this workout directly into your existing program (with the assumption that you have already warmed up).

Visual exercise reference

| Bird Dog | 160 |
| Reverse Curl | 156 |

Exercise Guide Note: execute the exercises in a controlled and smooth motion at a medium tempo. Perform all exercises consecutively, the completion of which constitutes one circuit. Complete two to three circuits (take a short rest if required), preferably without stopping.

CORE WORKOUT – REPETITION CIRCUITS
Workout 2
Workout difficulty: 2

Exercise	Reps	Circuits
Vacuum	2-3 Reps For Time (Count 15–20 Sec holds)	
Leg Passes	20 rotations	
Oblique Crunch	8–10 per side	
Side Plank/Reps	8–10 per side	
Climbing Twist	8–10 per side	
1 Circuit		2–3

When using as a standalone workout, include warm-up (five-to-ten-minutes), cool-down and stretch (four-to-five minutes). Warm-up time will be specific to your requirements and conditions. Cool-down and stretching time varies and depends on the stretch focus (maintenance or development). Read more on warm-up p.173, cool-down and stretching p.177. Alternatively, filter this workout directly into your existing program (with the assumption that you have already warmed up).

Visual exercise reference

Exercise Guide Note: execute the exercises in a controlled and smooth motion at a medium tempo. Perform all exercises consecutively, the completion of which constitutes one circuit. Complete two to three circuits (take a short rest if required), preferably without stopping.

CORE WORKOUT – REPETITION CIRCUITS
Workout 3
Workout difficulty: 3

Exercise	Reps	Circuits
Plank with Lateral Shift	30 shifts	
Leg Passes	20 rotations	
Jack-Knife Sit-Up	8–10	
Seated Row Crunch	15–20	

Side Plank with Twist	10–15 per side	
Reverse Curl	10–15	
Superman	10–15	
1 Circuit		2–4

When using as a standalone workout, include warm-up (five-to-ten-minutes), cool-down and stretch (four-to-five minutes). Warm-up time will be specific to your requirements and conditions. Cool-down and stretching time varies and depends on the stretch focus (maintenance or development). Read more on warm-up p.173, cool-down and stretching p.177. Alternatively, filter this workout directly into your existing program (with the assumption that you have already warmed up).

Visual exercise reference

Warm-up exercises	175
Seated Row Crunch	153
Plank with Lateral Shift	163
Side Plank with Twist	165
Leg Passes	170
Reverse Curl	156
Jack-Knife Sit-Up	169
Superman	166

Exercise Guide Note: execute the exercises in a controlled and smooth motion at a medium tempo. Perform all exercises consecutively, the completion of which constitutes one circuit. Complete two to four circuits (take a short rest if required), preferably without stopping.

CORE WORKOUT – REPETITION CIRCUITS
Workout 4
Workout difficulty: 3

Exercise	Reps	Circuits
Plank (Hold)	30–60 (Count 30–60 Sec Hold)	
Bicycle	20 rotations	
Russian Twist	8–10 per side	
V-UP Alternate	5–10 per side	
Oblique Crunch	10–15 per side	
Supine Bridge	10–15	
Crunch	10–15	
1 Circuit		2–4

When using as a standalone workout, include warm-up (five-to-ten-minutes), cool-down and stretch (four-to-five minutes). Warm-up time will be specific to your requirements and conditions. Cooldown and stretching time varies and depends on the stretch focus (maintenance or development). Read more on warm-up p.173, cooldown and stretching p.177. Alternatively, filter this workout directly into your existing program (with the assumption that you have already warmed up).

Visual exercise reference

Warm-up exercises	175
V-UP Alternate	168
Plank	161
Oblique Crunch	155
Bicycle	157
Supine Bridge	81
Russian Twist	158
Crunch	150

Exercise Guide Note: execute the exercises in a controlled and smooth motion at a medium tempo. Any (isometric) hold should be approached with full motor-unit contraction. Perform all exercises consecutively, the completion of which constitutes one circuit. Complete two-to-four circuits (take a short rest if required), preferably without stopping.

CORE WORKOUT – TIMED CIRCUITS
Workout 4
Workout difficulty: 3

Exercise	Time	Rest Between Circuits	Circuits
Plank (Hold)	30 Sec	30–45 Sec	
Leg Passes	30 Sec		
Climbing Twist	30 Sec		
Plank with Lateral Shift	30 Sec		

Superman	30 Sec		
Seated Row Crunch	30 Sec		
1 Circuit (3 minutes)			3–4

When using as a standalone workout, include warm-up (five-to-ten-minutes), cool-down and stretch (four-to-five minutes). Warm-up time will be specific to your requirements and conditions. Cool-down and stretching time varies and depends on the stretch focus (maintenance or development). Read more on warm-up p.173, cool-down and stretching p.177. Alternatively, filter this workout directly into your existing program (with the assumption that you have already warmed up).

Visual exercise reference

Exercise Guide Note: execute the exercises in a controlled and smooth motion at a medium tempo. Any (isometric) hold should be approached will full motor-unit contraction. Perform all exercise at 30-second intervals consecutively; the completion of all intervals constitutes one circuit (three minutes). Complete three to four circuits, resting 30–45 seconds between circuits (adjust the rest period according to your specific needs).

CORE WORKOUT – TIMED CIRCUITS
Workout 5
Workout difficulty: 3

Exercise	Time	Rest Between Circuits	Circuits
Single-Leg Hold (Left Leg)	30 Sec	30–45 Sec	
Single-Leg Hold (Right Leg)	30 Sec		
Plank with Raised Leg (Hold)	15 Sec per Leg Raise		
Seated Row–Crunch Hold	30 Sec		
Climbing Twist	30 Sec		
Alternate Superman	30 Sec		
1 Circuit (3 minutes)			3–4

When using as a standalone workout, include warm-up (five-to-ten-minutes), cool-down and stretch (four-to-five minutes). Warm-up time will be specific to your requirements and conditions. Cool-down and stretching time varies and depends on the stretch focus (maintenance or development). Read more on warm-up p.173, cool-down and stretching p.177. Alternatively, filter this workout directly into your existing program (with the assumption that you have already warmed up).

Visual exercise reference

Exercise Guide Note: execute the exercises in a controlled and smooth motion at a medium tempo. Any (isometric) hold should be approached with full motor-unit contraction. Perform all exercises at 30-second intervals consecutively; the completion of all intervals constitutes one circuit (three minutes). Complete three to four circuits, resting 30–45 seconds between circuits (adjust the rest period according to your specific needs).

CORE WORKOUT – TIMED CIRCUITS
Workout 6
Workout difficulty: 3

Exercise	Time	Rest Between Circuits	Circuits
Side Plank (Left Side on Hand)	30 Sec	30–45 Sec	
Side Plank (Right Side on Hand)	30 Sec		
Bicycle	30 Sec		
Seated Row Crunch	30 Sec		
Reverse Curl	30 Sec		
Superman	30 Sec		
1 Circuit (3 minutes)			3–4

When using as a standalone workout, include warm-up (five-to-ten-minutes), cool-down and stretch (four-to-five minutes). Warm-up time will be specific to your requirements and conditions. Cool-down and stretching time varies and depends on the stretch focus (maintenance or development). Read more on warm-up p.173, cool-down and stretching p.177. Alternatively, filter this workout directly into your existing program (with the assumption that you have already warmed up).

Visual exercise reference

Exercise Guide Note: execute the exercises in a controlled and smooth motion at a medium tempo. Any (isometric) hold should be approached with full motor-unit contraction. Perform all exercises at 30-second intervals consecutively; the completion of all intervals constitutes one circuit (three minutes). Complete three to four circuits, resting 30–45 seconds between circuits (adjust the rest period according to your specific needs).

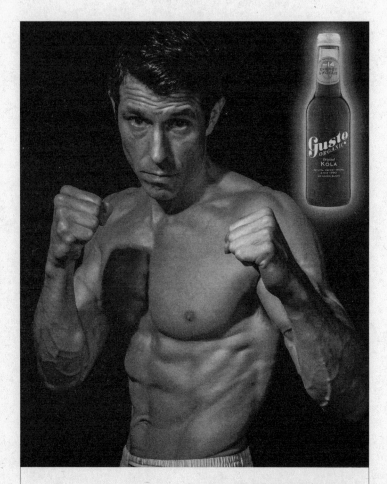

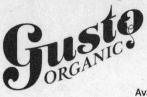